MUSIC, MOVEMENT, AND MIME
FOR CHILDREN

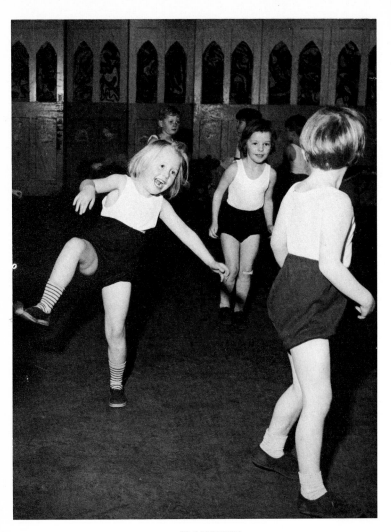

'PAULINE'

Music, Movement, and Mime for Children

VERA GRAY

AND

RACHEL PERCIVAL

LONDON
OXFORD UNIVERSITY PRESS

Oxford University Press, Ely House, London W. 1

GLASGOW   NEW YORK   TORONTO   MELBOURNE   WELLINGTON
CAPE TOWN   IBADAN   NAIROBI   DAR ES SALAAM   LUSAKA   ADDIS ABABA
DELHI   BOMBAY   CALCUTTA   MADRAS   KARACHI   LAHORE   DACCA
KUALA LUMPUR   SINGAPORE   HONG KONG   TOKYO

ISBN 0 19 317102 3

© Oxford University Press 1962

First published 1962
Seventh impression 1972

Printed in Great Britain

Preface

The battle for teaching young children Music and Movement at the same time was at its height in the nineteen-thirties and late forties, and no doubt there are still Resistance Groups simmering here and there. But by and large it is true to say that the battle has been won, and won as a direct result of BBC broadcasts initially inspired by the pioneer work of Ann Driver. It was primarily a battle to bring music of quality to young children in a way they could appreciate. As the authors of this book say, you can teach Movement successfully without any music at all, or with music that is not worth twopence. Even the great Laban, whose work on the movement side has been enormously influential even on those teachers who never heard of him, was willing to associate movement with improvised music of no lasting value. His methods were splendid for developing a child's sense of movement, but they scarcely helped his music at all. Music and Movement enthusiasts believe that you can teach Movement just as well in association with *good* music, and that you can *only* give young children a pleasurable awareness of simple musical facts in association with movement. To teach them together is in any case a great saving of time.

Those who hear Rachel Percival's excellent Music and Movement broadcasts week after week will already know a good deal about her work, though they will probably not know that it is Vera Gray who produces these programmes, chooses the music, and contributes a great deal to their success. A distinctive feature both of the programmes and of this book is the absence of imagery at the earlier stages. Young children, the authors believe, can only develop good movement to good music if they have nothing else to think about. Mime is of course valuable, but it is already sufficiently developed in other lessons at the Infant stage; in association with both movement and listening, it gives the younger children one thought-process more than they can cope with. In any case they are not likely at this stage to have either enough experience of life or a big enough repertoire of movement to make a proper job of miming to music. They will be ready to do this by the time they are Juniors, but not at the early Infant stage. It is the authors' experience that far better and more varied movement is obtained without imagery than with, and that this movement is much more free in that the children are less likely to imitate each other.

As a one-time member of the BBC's Schools Broadcasting Department, I was glad to read the description in this book of the long and arduous work that is put into the rehearsals for Music and Movement broadcasts. The belief that people who speak on the radio arrive in the studio five minutes before transmission with a few notes on the back of an envelope is not dead yet. (This did actually happen with certain music broadcasts for older children before the war, but it certainly does not happen nowadays.) There is mention in the pages that follow of the famous soloists who take part in these programmes and turn them into a musical experience that even the most brilliant teacher could not provide on her own. I remember one such player saying to me that it was less nerve-racking playing a concerto in the

Festival Hall than facing a Music and Movement script with a great deal crossed out, a great deal scribbled in (not always legibly), a sheet of music manuscript in a similar state of disorder, and a broadcaster liable to improvise something not in the script on transmission. But no hint of this strain ever seems to penetrate the microphone. All difficulties in the studio are regularly and triumphantly overcome.

But what of the difficulties in the classroom? The whole purpose of this book is to help teachers to surmount them. 'That ends today's recorded broadcast in the series, "Music and Movement",' says the announcer, and the teacher has only herself to rely on until the same time next week. This book gives advice on how to follow up the broadcasts, advice that can be understood by teachers with very few musical attainments or even with none at all. I do not myself believe that there is such a person as a teacher with no musical attainments, though there are many who lack confidence and think they have none. This is just the book to encourage and direct them. But more experienced teachers will also find new and stimulating ideas in these pages. Broadcasts may be able to provide musical experiences beyond the resources of any school, but they cannot be really successful without follow-up work by the teacher in-between-times. This book will help teachers to help their children towards fuller musical lives.

ROGER FISKE

CONTENTS

ILLUSTRATIONS

FOREWORD

Our collaboration on this book is an extension of the work prepared for the BBC programmes on Music and Movement.

As you will read in the chapter on 'The Broadcast' the programme is essentially dependent upon team work; Vera Gray is the musician and Rachel Percival the dancer.

If you are concerned about the relative importance of music or movement, we hope that the arrangement of the book will show that, in our experience, both subjects can be successfully taught together but at the same time each can be equally well developed on its own. There is no point in arguing whether one is more important than the other. The 'follow-up' chapter will provide some help towards developing the subject of your choice.

We have aimed at providing inexperienced *or* expert teachers with some material to build on or adapt as they wish.

VERA GRAY
RACHEL PERCIVAL

ACKNOWLEDGEMENTS

Grateful acknowledgement is due to the following for permission to reproduce photographs:

The British Broadcasting Corporation for frontispiece and fig. nos. 2, 3, 4, 5, 6, 7, 8, 9, 10, 20, 23, 30, 32, 35, 36, 37, 38 and 41 from St. Saviour's Infant School, Maida Vale, London, W.9 (Headmistress: Miss Kendall); and for fig. nos. 1, 13, 31, 39 and 40 from Horn Park Infant School, Alnwick Road, Lee (Headmistress: Miss Cocup).

Miss Burgess, Headmistress of Beverley Road Infant School, Chiswick, London, W.4, for fig. nos. 26, 28 and 29.

Mr. Tony Friese-Greene for fig. no. 21.

Miss Dorothy Simpson, M.B.E., and Mrs. E. Glyn for fig. nos. 11, 12, 18, 19, 22, 24, 25, 27, 33 and 34.

Miss E. Steiner, Warden of Children's Centre, Leeds 2, for fig. nos. 16 and 17.

Mr. H. Austin for fig. nos. 14 and 15.

Grateful acknowledgement is also due to Boosey & Hawkes, Music Publishers Ltd., for permission to quote from Bartok's *For Children*.

CHAPTER I

Movement

Music and movement have separate lives of their own, but in the beginning stages both can easily be taught together. They use the same words, they both need a creative approach, and preferably they should both have the same teacher. It is clearly impossible for an Infant teacher to be a specialist in every subject that she deals with during her crowded day; so, for the non-specialist, nervous of teaching movement, here are a few answers to the questions she may ask.

What is movement? Rudolf Laban's analysis is perhaps the simplest answer: every movement has a Time element, it takes place in Space, and it has a Weight element. So let us consider these elements separately before putting them together again to make a movement.

Time

A movement takes time. This can be short or long, depending on whether you move quickly or slowly. If you burn your fingers, you move away from danger as quickly as you can, but if you are threading a needle you move more slowly. Children hear the words 'quickly' and 'slowly' repeatedly from parents and teachers, in 'Come quickly' or 'Eat that slowly', and the difference between the words soon means something. In movement lessons for young children, it means moving very quickly contrasted with moving very slowly. Children enjoy these sudden changes of time.

> 'Run very fast.'
> 'Walk very slowly.'

> or

> 'Jump all over the floor quickly.'
> 'Sit down on the floor very slowly.'

At first it is easier for the young child to move quickly rather than slowly because a slow movement needs more control and co-ordination. It is more difficult to sit down slowly than to jump quickly, but if you alternate slow movements with quick, children will soon learn the difficult as well as the easy.

1. 'Make your feet dance high up in the air, quickly.'
2. 'Very slowly lift your leg up to the ceiling (—or 'in front of you', 'behind you', 'at the side of you').'
3. 'Let your feet dance all over the floor quickly.'
4. 'Slowly slide your feet along the floor: slide forwards, backwards and sideways slowly.'

Space

This is the Space Age. Children see and hear the word 'space' in 'Space Men', 'Space Suit', 'Space Rockets', and 'travelling through Space', and movements in space can be likened to this latest scientific development. Just as the rocket sets off from the earth into space so a movement can start from the body and lead out into space. As the rocket circles the moon so a movement can circle round the body. The large area of space surrounding the body can be divided into six zones: upper and lower; forward and backward; and left and right.

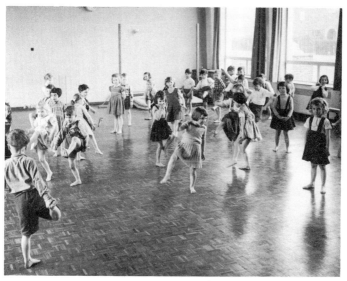

1   Lifting a leg up slowly—forwards, backwards, or sideways

Children use the space all round themselves happily at home, but quite often in school there is a teacher to be 'faced' which means that most movements are made in a forward direction. This is natural in the classroom; but in movement lessons it is a handicap. Children have to be encouraged to move in the space all round them.

1. 'Put your hand behind your back.

Look at your hand.
Now reach out as far as you can backwards.
See where your hand can lead you. It could move up
in the air, low down in front of you, or at the side.'

2. 'Kick forwards, backwards, sideways.'

3. 'Jump low down near the floor.
Jump high up in the air.
Jump round and round, high up in the air, and low
down near the floor.'

4. 'Slowly lift your leg up in front of you.
Slowly lift your leg up backwards, or sideways.
Lift your leg and step forwards, backwards, sideways,
and round and round.'

5. 'Slowly turn round and round.
Spin round quickly the other way.'

Floor, ceiling, and walls can be used to help the children
to direct their movement to a certain point.

1. 'Reach up to the ceiling.'
2. 'Stretch out to touch the walls.'
3. 'Punch down to the floor.'

The way to these targets can be *straight* or *twisted*. In other
words, the part of the body leading the movement may
draw a straight line or a more roundabout, twisted pattern.

1. 'Slowly grow up to the ceiling as straight as you can.'
2. 'Slowly curl and twist down to the floor again.'
By changing the time element you can build up a series of

movements based on a straight and twisted line directed to certain points.

1. 'Quickly move straight to the ceiling or walls; slowly twist back again down to the floor.'

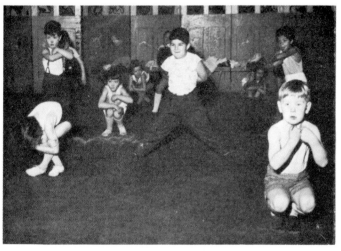

2 'Twist yourself into a knot'

2. 'Slowly move straight to the ceiling; twist back again down to the floor quickly.'

As children like sudden changes of time from very quick to very slow, so they enjoy changes of bodily shape from one extreme to another, such as shrinking into a narrow, closed-in position and growing out into a wide, open position. This can be done quickly or slowly; or alternating quick and slow, as in:

1. 'Make yourself very *thin* quickly; slowly grow out very *wide*.'
2. 'Slowly make yourself very *small*; grow up very *big* quickly.'
3. '*Twist* yourself into a knot, quickly.'
4. 'Slowly make yourself as *straight* as you can.'

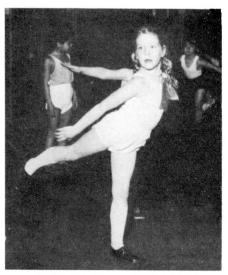

3   'Make yourself as straight as you can'

The three levels of movement make further divisions of space. These levels are: High (up on the toes); Medium (standing height); and Low (near the floor). When a whole class dances in a hall, rising and falling through these three levels, the effect can be quite spectacular.

'See if you can touch the floor and the ceiling as you dance slowly up and down, all over the room.'

By naming the level of the movement which you want the children to use, you can add extra zest and variety. If you preface a jump with 'Jump high in the air and then low down on the floor' it sounds simple enough but turns out to be quite difficult to do, and children are absorbed in their attempts.

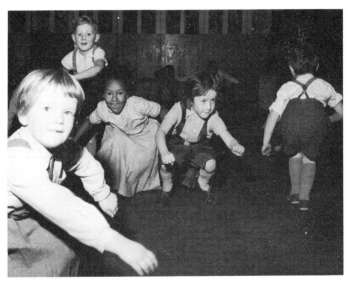

4 'Move low down near the floor'

Weight

Some of us may worry about our weight but even if we are heavy, it does not necessarily follow that we move heavily. Big people are often light on their feet. The quality of weight used in a movement is decided by the degree of tension used in the muscles. The word 'tension' stares down at us from advertisements; tranquillizers are prescribed to relieve exaggerated tension so that we can relax and feel 'lighter'. But these are for tired adults only. Through such movements as kicking, punching, and pressing, contrasted with smooth, gentle movements like gliding and floating, children will soon learn the difference between strong and light.

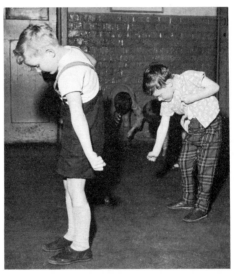

5 Punching

1. 'Punch down to the floor quickly.'
2. 'Lift your arms up slowly and gently.'

So the three elements of Time, Space, and Weight combine to produce movement qualities. The child can be taught to move quickly and slowly, strongly and lightly, in a straight and twisted fashion. The child can learn *how* to move and *where* to move. At the same time he can learn *what* parts of the body can move. The head, shoulders, elbows, knees, chin, chest, wrists, hips, fingers, side, back, and feet can lead a movement. This *body awareness* should be a constant theme throughout Infant lessons to encourage every child to move his whole body.

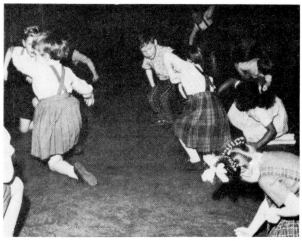

6 Leading up to the ceiling with an elbow, in preparation for an up-and-down dance

1. 'Curl up as small as you can.
   Slowly let your elbow go right up the ceiling.
   Curl up again quickly.'

2. 'This time let your chin or ear go up to the ceiling;
   your chin *or* ear.'

3. 'Slap your knees hard.
   Lift your knee as high as you can.
   Dance with your knees up to your chin.'

4. 'Put your elbow on your knee.
   Slowly lift your elbow away from your knee, as far
   away as you can.
   Put your elbow back on your knee, quickly.'

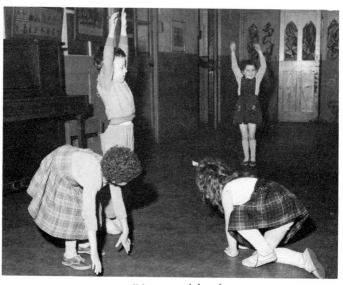

7   'Move up and down'

Locomotion

Moving from one spot to another is called 'locomotion'
and the most common form of this is running or walking.
When children are set free in a hall or playground, they run
around. From this natural reaction you can interest them in
the many other ways by which they can get from place to
place. All intricate steps in dance are made from the elementary steps of walking, running, leaping, hopping, jumping,
skipping, galloping, striding, and sliding.

These steps can all be done in many different ways if you experiment with the elements which make them 'elementary', on the lines mentioned above, alternating quick and slow time, with straight or twisted directions in space, using a strong or light weight.

Children will often invent unusual ways of locomotion

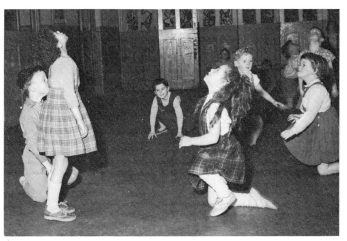

8   Chins leading up to the ceiling

for themselves, like walking on all fours, on their hands or knees, rolling over and over, or somersaulting. If you are at hand to suggest stressing different elements—'can you do that slowly?' or 'try moving in a straight line like that'—you can open up new channels for the child's own invention to explore.

Shape

If we could see the patterns of human movements in the

air (as we can see jet trails) we would realize the wide range of possible shapes. Shapes can be 'drawn' in space by many different parts of the body and some shapes can be formed by the body itself. The basic shapes are a straight line, a circle or curve, a twisted pattern, and an angle; each shape can be

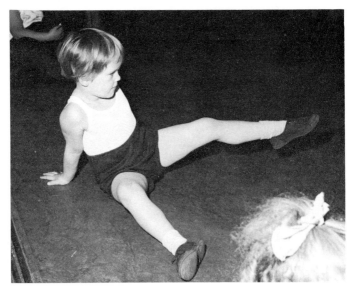

9   Drawing a straight line with a foot

drawn by finger, hand, arm, elbow, head, foot, knee, or leg. Different sizes can be drawn: ask the children to draw a small circle, then a bigger and still bigger one. Numbers or letters provide ready-made shapes to draw, in a series of suggestions like:

1. 'Write a figure two on the floor.'
2. 'Write it as small as you can.'

3. 'Write a figure two as large as you can in the air.'
4. 'Try writing a figure two on the ceiling.'
5. 'Now write it at the side of you.'

Again, changing the Time and Weight elements will give a new look to a familiar movement.

1. 'Draw a figure three quickly and lightly.'

Discipline in Movement

You may think that with such freedom there can be no discipline, but the task is itself a discipline if the movement qualities are experienced to the full. The simple movement of running quickly and stopping abruptly will encourage self-control in children as well as amuse them. Think of the fun of 'musical chairs' or 'statues'! You can make this training more exciting and help to develop movement at the same time if you stop the children high up in the air or low down near the floor, in various positions, straight and twisted. Next ask for a movement which ends gradually: this needs sustained control and will help to quieten a class, for a child must listen very carefully to follow music from quick to slow to stop.

Children seem to take it for granted that they are likely to be knocked down, bumped into, and tripped up in school. Movement lessons can teach them to avoid many a rough-and-tumble, for they must learn to use their eyes to find a space to dance in and they must learn control of their feet to dodge round other children in a crowded hall.

Group Work

When adults think of 'dancing' they usually think of dancing with somebody, and the social side often outweighs the technical. Children, too, enjoy dancing with somebody or in a group. As they learn to avoid collisions, and to stop and start together, children become conscious of other children dancing in the same hall at the same time. This consciousness leads on to work in smaller groups who may dance together with a leader playing a percussion instrument, or even to work with partners. Infant days are early for young children to dance together, but at least movement lessons will emphasize the 'give-and-take' that you encourage throughout the day.

Summary

To sum up, here are the ten points of departure for movement education in the Infant school:

1.	Body awareness:	Any part of the body can start a movement: head, shoulders, elbows, knees, back, wrists, hips, chest, chin, eyes, ears, feet, arms, hands, sides, and fingers.
2.	Variation of Time:	Quick; slow.
3.	Use of Space:	Directions: towards floor, ceiling, and walls. Straight and twisted movements. Extensions: narrow to wide movements.
4.	Levels:	High, medium, and low.
5.	Use of Weight:	Strong, heavy, and light.
6.	Locomotion:	Walking; leaping; running; hopping; jumping; skipping; galloping; and striding.

7. Flow: Sudden or gradual stops.

8. Shape formation: Lines, circles, angles, and figures-of-eight, drawn in the air or on the floor. Shapes made by the body itself, rounded, angular, or twisted.

9. Group Work: Beginning to dance in small groups or with a partner.

10. All possible combinations of these.

Once on the way, these two points should travel with you:

1. *How* you move to a position is as important as getting there. Whether you move quickly or slowly, straight or twisted, strongly or lightly, you can only encourage the beginnings of a dance technique by suggesting the different 'hows' repeatedly.

2. You can only develop from the random and slapdash by realizing this: large, vigorous, and exhausting movements are not the sole aim of a movement lesson: small, delicate movements are just as valuable if the children are concentrating.

CHAPTER II

Music and Movement

All aspects of music can have their beginnings in the association of music with movement. In this work music is in no way subordinate.

To many teachers music may seem, in some respects, to be beyond their powers. However, these days there are so many simply-used percussion and melodic instruments, as well as records, that the teacher with little musical knowledge and no ability to play the piano can easily give young children the beginnings of a musical training. In the following material, examples will show how a teacher could improvise music for various movements.

Chapter I shows how movement is expressed in terms of Time, Weight, and Space. These three terms can very well be applied to music.

Time

As movement can be expressed in terms of time, i.e. quick and slow, so can music. A tune can be either quick or slow. Here is a fast tune to which children could run quickly:

Fig. 1.

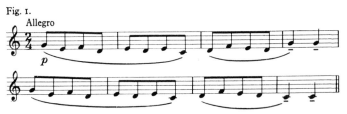

This piece of music is by Bartók and is from *For Children*, Vol. I, No. 4. It is a very simple tune and the teacher can easily sing it to 'lah', play it on a recorder, chime bars, or dulcimer, or with one hand on the piano. It can be tapped rhythmically on a tambour, or of course the recording can be used. Nursery rhymes can also be used very effectively. Some examples of quick running tunes are:

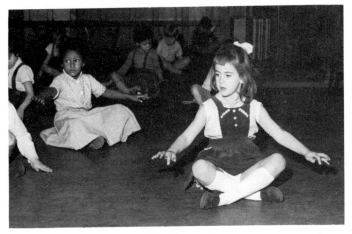

10   Tapping to music

Bobby Shafto
Yankee Doodle
Polly Flinders
Polly Put the Kettle On.

Musical terms giving clues to the speed of the music can be found at the top left-hand corner of the first line. Here are some of the commonest terms used indicating quick speed: allegro; vivace; presto; prestissimo; vivo or vif;

volante. (See Appendix C.) For those who are quite unable to read music, an even, regular, quick beat on a tambour will set the rhythmic quality for a running movement. For other quick movements the actual words of the movement, regularly grouped, will give the rhythmic pattern:

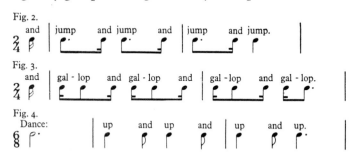

Fig. 2.
Fig. 3.
Fig. 4.

Once the words have set the rhythm, the pattern can then be taken over on the tambour.

Music can also be slow. Slow music and slow movements need a greater degree of control and concentration than quick music and movements. Here again the same range of

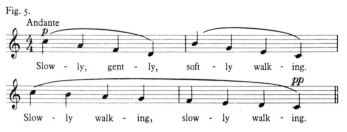

Fig. 5.

instruments can be used as for the quick movements. Indications of slow music are: lento or lente; adagio; andante; largo; larghetto; maestoso. (See Appendix C.) A tune like the one in Fig. 5, based on a bell pattern, can be fun. Words can be fitted to it, but it is important that the quality which is required in the movement should be suggested by the character of the singing and the words which are chosen. In Fig. 5, the words, 'Slowly, gently, softly walking' should be sung in such a way that the children will correctly interpret the mood. Here the sustained quality is indicated by the slur over the notes. The soft indications are shown also in this example—*p* meaning soft and *pp* very soft. Some nursery rhymes for slow movement are:

> I Love Little Pussy
> Lavender's Blue
> Dance a Baby Diddy
> Curly Locks.

A further step in Time is a *gradual* increase of speed from slow to quick. Children more easily recognize this than music decreasing in pace. In Fig. 6 the quickening pace is indicated by the word accelerando and slackening of pace by the word ritardando. Other words which might have been used are, for quickening: stringendo; for slackening: rallentando, ritenuto or allargando. (See Appendix C.) These examples show the use that can be made of scale passages and notes of the key chord.

Time is best presented to young children by means of contrast. The words 'quick' and 'slow' must be stressed:

> e.g. 'Dance as *quickly* as this music.'
> 'Walk as *slowly* as this music.'

The activities in a lesson based on time should be given in these contrasted terms.

Fig. 6.

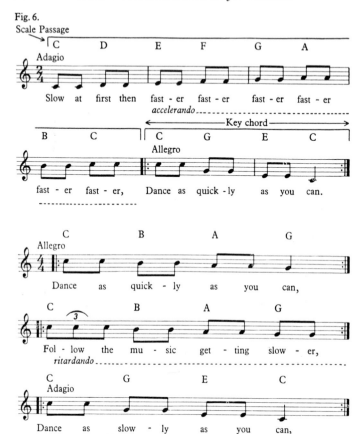

The tune may be sung to 'lah' when the music is repeated, as in bars 5 & 6 of the first example and each bar of the second.

Already in the previous examples characteristics other than Time have been present. In fact, both music and movement are composed of a combination of qualities. Another of these is Weight.

Weight

Weight in music, in its simplest form, is conveyed by loudness and softness. Strength in movement can be allied to loud music; gentleness and lightness of movement to soft music. As you have read in Chapter I, strong movements are varied. They can be strong and slow (e.g. pressing feet into the ground), or strong and quick (e.g. punching). Figs. 7 and 8 below show this in music. The children will recognize that Fig. 7 is again a very simple bell pattern and Fig. 8 makes use of the tune of a nursery rhyme 'The Keel Row'. The

Fig. 7.

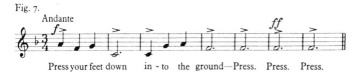

Press your feet down in - to the ground—Press. Press. Press.

Fig. 8.

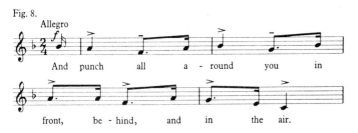

And punch all a - round you in front, be - hind, and in the air.

teacher's use of such material may encourage the children to make up their own music and words for movement.

In using examples of this kind it is important that the strength of the movement comes through. Well-articulated words and strong rhythms will convey the mood.

In addition to the above type of vocal improvisation, effective instrumental music can be played on gongs, cymbals, large tambours, or drums, if these are available. Padded or hard sticks can be used according to the quality of the sound required. Indications of loudly accented music can be seen in Figs. 7 and 8 by the marks above the notes (– or >), the second mark being stronger than the first. In some music the word 'marcato' is printed underneath if every note has to be accented. Loud and very loud is shown by the abbreviations *f* or *ff*. (See Appendix C.) Nursery tunes suggesting strength include:

> Aiken Drum
> Oranges and Lemons
> Dr. Foster.

Gentleness and lightness in music are often associated with a quick pace as shown in Fig. 1, but they can also be combined with a slow pace as in Fig. 2. Nursery tunes which suggest a light or gentle quality are:

> My Lady's Garden
> Curly Locks
> Lavender's Blue
> Lady Bird.

These nursery rhymes can be found in *The Oxford Nursery Song Book* (see Appendix B). Common musical indications of these qualities are the abbreviations *p* and *pp* and the words dolce (sweetly), leggiero (lightly), and grazia (gracefully). (See Appendix C.) Instruments which are particularly suitable for suggesting light qualities of sound are chime bars, Indian bells, and triangles (played lightly); the tambour, tambourine, or drum (played with padded sticks or the fingers); and the temple blocks (which give a hollow, light sound). Children should be given the opportunity to experiment with these instruments in order to experience the making of sounds of different weight.

Weight in music is more easily understood by the children when it is presented in terms of contrast, e.g. 'Punch as strongly as you can to the *loud* music and dance as gently and lightly as you can to the *soft* gentle music.' An extension of this is the gradual change from one to the other: from light to strong and from strong to light movements. This is commonly expressed in music by the terms crescendo or ——————— and diminuendo or ——————. This can be done effectively by a 'shimmer' on a cymbal or a roll on a drum.

Space

The way in which a melody moves in music is allied to Space in movement. There are two aspects of this to consider. Movements are made at different levels—high, medium, and low—and in music we can have high, medium, and low notes. This is called *pitch* in music. Here is an example of a tune moving from high to low notes to which the children could be asked to jump high and low.

Fig. 9.

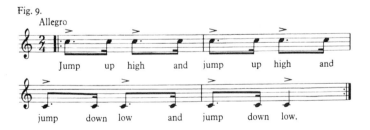

Young children have difficulty in distinguishing between these levels of pitch, so they should not be burdened with the decision as to whether the tune is high or low. A way of teaching pitch to children can be found in Chapter V.

Effective percussion instruments for high and low notes could be Indian bells, triangles, or jingle bells alternating with tambour or drum. Fig. 9 shows a vocal line using top doh and bottom doh to indicate contrasted levels. Even those who do not play the piano will find that the black notes used alone will give a pleasant tune in whatever order they are played. Single notes or chords on the black notes, making use of the whole range of the keyboard, will provide suitable music for gradual changes of movement from low to high, e.g.:

1. 'Curl up as small as you can as the music gets lower.' *Piano*. Choose *one* black note, e.g. F♯, and play it in octaves, starting at the top of the treble and moving to the bass. Use both hands and keep the right pedal down.
2. 'Grow up as high as you can as the music gets higher.' *Piano*. As for 1. but start in the bass and move up to the top of the treble.

Another aspect of melody is the direction in which it moves. Some tunes move in a direct or straight fashion like the nursery rhyme: 'Upon Paul's Steeple'.

Fig. 10.

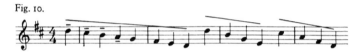

Others are indirect and curl and twist like 'Curly Locks'.

Fig. 11.

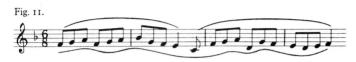

'Hot Cross Buns' is an example of a tune which moves in a straight and in a curling fashion.

Fig. 12.

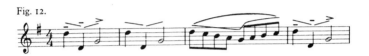

Locomotion

A single repeated note is suitable for movement on the spot, while melody can be the signal for dancing all over the room.

Fig. 13.

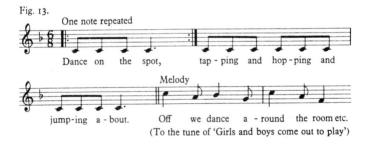

(To the tune of 'Girls and boys come out to play')

Useful Rhythms

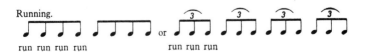

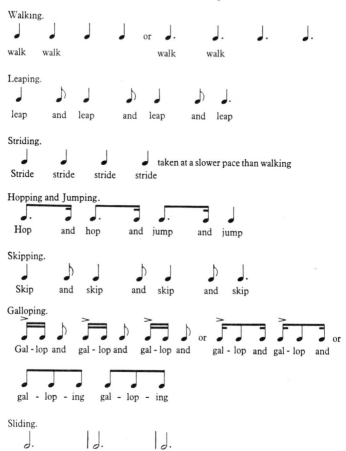

Children should be encouraged to use percussion instruments in the music and movement lesson. The teacher can at first give practice in the use of instruments in the classroom when children are grouped around her for music making. Individual children could play instruments to which the rest of the class could move, e.g.:

'Shake your hands hard when John plays the jingle bells.'
'Nod your head when you hear Pat's sticks.' (Pat could have rhythm sticks.)
'Make as many different straight shapes as you can when Polly plays the cymbals.' (Polly could clash the cymbals together.)
'Curl and twist your hands as John shakes the tambourine.'

The teacher could lead this by playing herself and then handing over to a child. In this way the whole class would become familiar with the use of percussion instruments and their sounds and would find no strangeness in using them in the music and movement lessons. Individual children or a group could set a musical pattern for all to move to. The teacher can discuss with the class the instruments that would

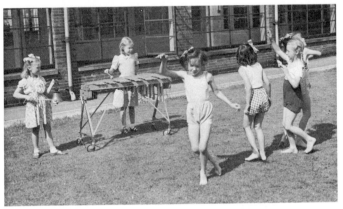

11 Playing for a dance made up by a group of children in their free time
(without the teacher present)

best suit the movement, the children giving the suggestions and the teacher guiding their choice: several instruments may be suggested and used at the same time for one movement. In this way an orchestrated effect can be obtained. Interesting group work can be done with one group working

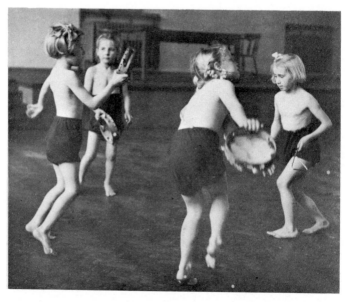

12   Four girls making up a dance together, using three tambourines and one triangle

in contrast to the other. One or more of each group could have percussion instruments. In a lesson where the stress is on weight, and the contrast is in light and strong music and movement, the light group could work with Indian bells and maracas while the contrasting group could work with clashing cymbals and tambourines hit with the palm of the hand. The instrumentalists can move with their group or work as a band at the side of the room.

The interest in making music in this way will be intensified if the children have made their own percussion instruments. Further information on music-making is given in Chapter V.

Percussion Instruments Commonly Found in Schools:
  Drum and Tambour
These can be played with the fingers, hand, hard or padded sticks, or a wire brush. Hard sticks are generally available and a padded stick can easily be made by covering the top of a piece of thin rod with first a piece of foam rubber and then circular pieces of soft material (e.g. lint) gathered around the edges and drawn up tightly. A wire brush can be made from a piece of electric cable about 8 inches long. Fray out 4 inches of the cable, and leave the remaining 4 inches to serve as the handle. A great variety of sounds are possible from the drum and tambour, varying according to the way in which they are struck and whether the hand or a stick is used. For example, for slow walking play either a drum or a tambour with a padded stick using slow, even beats; for quick running play one of these instruments with either the tips of the fingers or lightly with a hard stick, using quick, even beats.

  The Tambourine
Because of the jingles attached to the instrument it can be shaken as well as struck. It can be played with the hand, hard sticks, or padded sticks. The shake can vary in intensity and can accompany a movement such as, 'As the tambourine gets softer make yourself as thin as you can.' Alternations of

soft and loud shaking could be used for moving in a twisted fashion, for example: 'Run in a twisted line all over the floor.'

Pairs of Cymbals

These can be struck together either quickly or slowly, loudly or softly. A series of sharp clashes could be interpreted by a movement such as, 'Shoot out your arms and legs quickly all round you.' A series of slow, soft clashes would set the music for slow pointing with hands, feet, and elbows in various directions.

A single cymbal can be held by the leather handle or suspended on a stand and hit with either a padded stick, a hard stick or even a wire brush. For light movements it is best to hit the cymbal with the padded stick or wire brush; a hard stick, however it is used, makes a very brittle noise on the cymbal and should be used sparingly. A roll on the cymbal with a padded stick is very effective for heavy twisted movements, and crescendo and decrescendo rolls for movements which involve gaining or losing strength. Hitting the cymbal at the end of a roll will suggest climax and terminate a movement.

The school percussion band rarely has a large cymbal and it is advisable to add a twelve-inch instrument, which sounds much richer for use with movement.

The Triangle

A triangle can be struck slowly on the horizontal bar to make single notes that can either be cut short by damping the sound with the fingers holding the triangle, or left sounding. For quick movement the beater can be moved rapidly in the angle nearest the open end of the instrument.

The Gong

This is hit with a padded stick. Rapid hitting can give a sustained sound and can be effective if coupled with crescendo or diminuendo. The gong could be struck at regular intervals for a movement such as pressing the feet heavily into the floor or for striding.

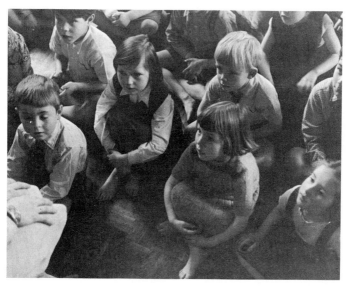

13 Listening to music

Bells

Bells mounted on either end of a stick can be used for a light, quick movement. When shaken they can be used for either continuous or intermittent sound.

Indian Bells

These tiny 'cymbals' have a sweet quality of sound. The

ring is not so urgent as that of the triangle. The bells are tapped together and the sound can either be left to ring or be stopped by touching the bells with the fingers.

Rhythm Sticks

These are either pairs of coloured sticks or flat pieces of wood with handles, which can be hit together and used for light direct movements, quick or slow.

Melodic Percussion Instruments
Chime Bars, Dulcimer, and Tubular Bells

A whole set of chime bars consisting of two octaves can be obtained, but this is costly. They can be acquired singly, and it would be wise to build a set of notes that would be useful for all kinds of work, for melody-making in the classroom as well as for use with movement. Certain notes will give a pleasant tune, no matter in what order they are struck: C D E G A. These are the notes of the pentatonic scale. (See Chapter V.) The sound of the chime bar is not suitable for strong movements but would be very effective for light and gentle movements, whether quick or slow. The dulcimer is not so resonant as chime bars and can be used for light, quick movements. Tubular bells can be made from old brass curtain rods, but care must be taken to get the tubes filed down to the right length to give a true set of notes.

Other Useful Percussion Instruments
Whip

This can be made by hinging a shorter piece of wood on to a longer piece—the extra piece of wood making a handle.

The sound is most effective when movements are spasmodic, quick, and strong, e.g.: 'When you hear the whip, shoot out an arm or a leg.'

Temple Blocks or Skulls
Old temple blocks can sometimes be picked up for very little money in second-hand shops. They vary in size and so in sound, and can be played with wooden or rubber-headed

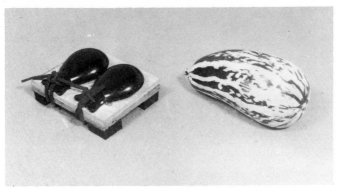

14   Castanets attached to a sheet of asbestos by means of thick rubber strips. A painted, dried gourd, filled with pearl-barley and used as a maraca

sticks. They can be used for light direct movements, quick or slow.

Maracas
These can be made by partly filling cardboard cylinders with dried peas or rice. They are effective when shaken and are used for quick movements.

Castanets
These can be very difficult to play in the Spanish way,

but can be easily manipulated on a wooden block. To make this, screw the base of one castanet to a block and attach the other half by strong rubber through the normal holes. Any rhythm can then very easily be played.

Wooden Tapping Block
This is hit with wooden-headed sticks and is used for

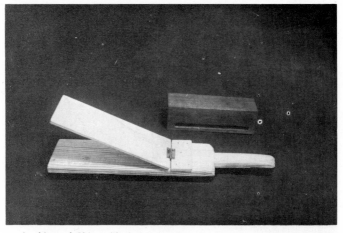

15   A whip, and Chinese block showing the side of the instrument with the slot in the wood which is cut almost through to the other side. There is a corresponding slot on the other side. The block must be made of hard wood

quick, light, and straight movements. (Thimbles worn on first and second fingers of the right hand make a good substitute for sticks.)

NOTE: a percussion trolley would make the transport of all these instruments from classroom to hall an easy operation.

String and Wind Instruments
Other orchestral instruments, including the piano, are

welcome in movement lessons only if they can be played well. They can all be used together with or in contrast to percussion, as most of them can play for all kinds of movement, whether straight or twisted, strong, light, quick, or slow. Teacher and accompanist should, however, decide well beforehand exactly how the music is to be played, so that tempo, expression, and the shaping of the musical phrases are agreed on. No two musicians ever interpret the same piece in quite the same way and yet both may be obeying the instructions in the music.

Without all these instruments one can still make a variety of rhythmical patterns and sounds with voice, hands and feet. Hands and feet are themselves very effective instruments. Clapping with hands alternately cupped then outstretched provides heavy and light sound. Finger-snapping is light and foot-stamping is heavy. Alternations of these light and heavy sounds will give control of weight. They can be used quickly and slowly.

CHAPTER III

Music, Movement, and Mime

Children love to act and they need no stage or audience to encourage them. They can be cowboys yelling, 'Hi-yo, Silver', or scientists counting, 'Five, four, three, two, one, zoom', in playground, classroom, or corridor. As for dancing, all they want is freedom, space, and the chance to be something or somebody else. There is, however, this clear distinction between dance and drama: in dance, the child is expressing himself; in drama, he expresses the character he is playing. For a brief space of time he *is* a cowboy, and his movements and speech belong to the cowboy. If children have a rich store of movements to draw on, their interpretations will be original and not copied from someone else. So let the children have plenty of time to experiment in movement. If this experimental period is denied them, the children, wanting to please the teacher, will copy the first child to move and will not think for themselves. Teachers can also point out through poems, songs, stories, and pictures that there are many ways of being a fairy, a giant, or a dwarf, and so avoid building up such a cliché as arm-waving which passes equally for a fairy, a tree, a butterfly, and an aeroplane.

There are eight basic effort actions or expressive movements which are built up from the three elements of Time,

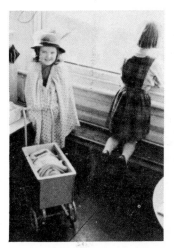

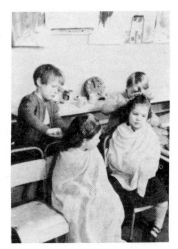

16 Four-year-olds playing at mothers and babies in the house

17 Three- and four-year-olds playing at hair-dressing

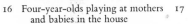

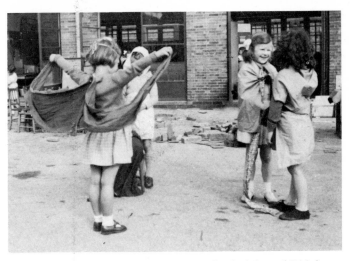

18 Six-year-olds in spontaneous dramatic play, 'Witches and Fairies', with improvised dressing-up clothes from old pieces of material

Space, and Weight, and whose names may give a clue to a possible character:

1. Punching: quick, straight, and strong
2. Pressing: slow, straight, and strong
3. Wringing: slow, twisted, and strong
4. Slashing: quick, twisted, and strong
5. Flicking: quick, twisted, and light
6. Floating: slow, twisted, and light
7. Dabbing: quick, straight, and light
8. Gliding: slow, straight, and light.

A combination of these movements can suggest a story. A powerful king might Punch, Press, and Slash, a beautiful princess Float, Glide, and Dab, and the wicked witch Wring her hands as she schemes. An unending supply of characters can be created from these expressive movements. You can ask the children, 'What person would punch?' and they may answer a soldier, cowboy, policeman, or little boy in the playground. The answers to, 'Who is he punching?' and, 'Why is he punching?' will give the basis of a story. The policeman may be attacked by a robber who is escaping through a wood. What happens in the wood, who and what they meet there, and whether the policeman catches the robber should give you a great deal of action as well as detail.

Keep these eight possibilities constantly in mind so that there is no danger of a character being typed. For instance, a calm 'gliding' witch who suddenly 'slashes' may be much more effective in some situations than the more usual 'curling' and 'twisting' variety. In fact, there are times when a witch could profitably Punch, Press, Wring, Slash, Flick, Float, Dab, *and* Glide.

The simple movements of locomotion can be another basis for mime.

1. 'Walk very slowly as if you were tired.'
2. 'Now walk up a big hill.'
3. 'Run down the other side of this big hill.'
4. 'Now you're walking on ice; be careful not to slip down.'
5. 'This time, you're carrying something . . . perhaps a heavy sack . . . or a pint of milk.'
6. 'You walk on two legs. What walks on four legs?' (A cow, horse, dog, elephant, lion, tiger, donkey, etc.) 'You walk on four legs like a (chosen animal).'
7. 'Are you walking on grass? In a wood? On the road? On the sand? And are you in a hurry? How old are you? Very old? Or very young?'

The remaining methods of locomotion—leaping, hopping, jumping, skipping, galloping, striding, and their combinations—can be used in a similar way.

Things which children have seen can lead to more suggestions. 'What did you see on your way to school? Roadsweeper? Builder? Road mender? Postman?' The working actions of these men can be mimed by the children and, with your help, they can feel as if they are really doing the job. Your help amounts to working out an analysis of the action in Time, Space, and Weight, taking into consideration the nature of the job, the tools used, what clothes are worn and the age of the person. For example if the road sweeper is sweeping leaves, his movements will probably be lighter than if he were sweeping mud. Suppose he was sweeping mud: he would move the brush slowly, in a straight line, using a great deal of strength, which is, in fact, a Pressing movement along the ground. For sweeping leaves he would probably use less strength so that the movement would be nearer to a Glide than a Press.

When children do imaginary sweeping, they usually clench their fists tightly and perform some sort of swinging movement causing the imaginary dust to fly in the air. Remind them that they are holding a wooden handle and that the dirt has to be kept on the floor. In other words, make the mime as accurate as possible.

We all enjoy seeing the actor on the stage or in films eating real food and drinking real liquid of some kind—even if it is only cold tea instead of whisky—and although this may not be practical in school, the children can have great fun in pretending to eat and drink. More fun can be had if you see that they eat and drink realistically by asking them what they are eating, whether it needs a lot of chewing and whether they like it. This is where we return to the eight basic effort actions done in miniature. Imagine *Pressing* your teeth into an apple, or the *Wringing* movement of trying to extricate toffee from top and bottom teeth, the *Dabbing* movement of eating nuts or the *Gliding* of ice-cream licking. You need not necessarily use these movement terms with the young children but could get the same result by introducing one element at a time.

1. 'Pretend you have an ice-cream cornet.
   Lick your ice-cream slowly.'

2. 'Lick your ice-cream very gently and lightly.'
3. 'Lick your ice-cream slowly and gently.'
4. 'Lick it straight or you will lose it.'

Places which children have visited can give you other ideas for mime. Visits to the zoo, circus, or fairground could have many possibilities, especially if the visits are backed up with stories, poems, and actual facts. Here again, truth must go hand-in-hand with imagination; just walking on four legs will not do for *all* four-footed animals. Rabbits jump from the back two legs on to the front two legs. Horses, cows, and dogs have a much more complicated sequence of movements: for galloping they stretch out their front two legs forwards, the back two legs stretch out backwards and then both pairs meet in the middle. When walking, they move first a front leg and then a back leg on the opposite side. Elephants and camels move two legs on the same side then the two legs on the other side. Sparrows do not hop but jump on two feet, and ducks stand on one leg. Imitating the movement qualities of birds and animals can widen the range of children's movements. The heaviness of an elephant contrasted with the lightness of a sparrow will give a new experience in movement and mime to a child.

With this kind of mime, you can play a game in which the class guesses what animals are being imitated. Guessing like this will put both the performers and the class watching on their mettle and sharpen up their movement observation.

Next you could ask how they went to the zoo or circus. This can lead on to various kinds of transport such as buses, boats and aeroplanes. The use of different levels and speeds can help to distinguish each machine as in high levels for aeroplanes, middle for buses, and low for boats.

Mimes like these have all been based on what the class has *seen* or *done* but imaginary stories and poems can be just as useful. Every child can act each part as you tell the story, or each part can be acted by groups of children, or a combination of individuals and groups can give a more detailed interpretation.

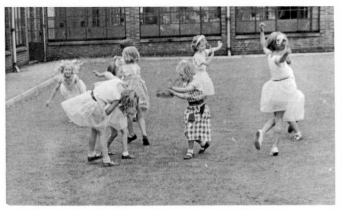

19   Dance made up by Nina (with tambourine). Originally a pure dance
with Nina as a leader; the dressing-up was an afterthought

Broad interpretation of a story

In most fairy stories you have the good character (fairy godmother), the bad (witch or giant), the funny (clown or dwarf), and the law (king or father). Working in these four groups you can make up your own fairy story. For example, the good fairies are being entertained by the clowns (perhaps accompanied by or playing tambourines and castanets), the bad witches enter to the sound of drums and cymbals, the clowns run away and the good fairies are frightened. The witches dance triumphantly not knowing that the clowns have gone to tell the king about the fight. The king and his soldiers arrive and drive the witches away. The witches then promise to be good so the king allows them to come back and everyone dances together at the end.

Working in more detail, use a familiar story and let all the children have the chance to do what they think each character would do before you choose one child for any particular part. In choosing, remember the danger of cliché, and look occasionally for the unorthodox to encourage children to invent rather than recall other interpretations they may have seen.

Combination of broad and detailed interpretation

Traditional fairy tales can be tailor-made for top classes in the Infant School. 'The Sleeping Beauty', for example, gives opportunity for group work and for individual parts. The cast includes the princess, the good fairies, the bad fairy, the king and queen, the palace staff, and the prince. Tragedy strikes when the bad fairy casts a wicked spell over the baby princess. She may do this in many different ways:

1. She might mingle with the crowds unseen, then suddenly slash her way through to the baby princess to shout her curse.
2. She might appear, slowly glide forward—building up tension gradually—and then pronounce her curse as the climax.
3. She might dance in happily and gleefully, stop suddenly, slowly point to the child, and then speak.

Meanwhile the rest of the party can react in their own ways. The queen may be rooted to the spot, with her mouth open but unable to speak; she could faint; or she could even try to get to the baby princess. The king could try to stop the bad fairy; he could hold his head in horror; or he may call his guards to act. The courtiers, good fairies and servants might tremble, close their eyes, protest, or be struck dumb with fear. Authority speaks when the king banishes all spinning wheels from the palace:

1. The king can be a forceful character who stamps and rages, forbidding all spinning wheels.
2. He could be calm but still strong as he makes his pronouncement in a dignified manner.
3. He could panic and fuss in and out of every room, making sure that all the spinning wheels had been thrown away.

Humour can be introduced when the whole palace full of people go to sleep in the middle of whatever they are doing. The cook may be tasting his soup, the kitchen boy peeling vegetables, the gardener digging potatoes, the chambermaid making the beds, the butler pouring drinks, and the queen yawning. In fact this brings us back to working actions once more, but here the children stop in the middle of their working actions, like statues. A happy ending allows everyone a chance to take part in a dance when the prince wakes the princess and marries her.

Poetry
Poems like 'The Owl and the Pussycat' by Edward Lear

could be mimed by a small group while the rest of the class speaks the words. With your knowledge of Time, Space, and Weight, you can help the children to get meaningful expression into their speech.

Suspense can be produced by slow speech gradually accelerating to quick. When Red Riding Hood tells her grandmother (who is really the wolf) what big teeth she has, the wolf may answer first slowly, then quickly, 'All the better to gobble you up, my dear,' and Red Riding Hood will be truly frightened.

Voices on one level may be more menacing than voices which soar through the three levels.

'Come here, come here,' spoken on one level only and, 'I haven't done anything wrong,' spoken through three levels, high, medium and low, can immediately give you the different characters of these two people.

Light, sweet-voiced characters often come up against strong, gruff-voiced characters in stories and poems. The strong, direct voice usually frightens while the light, flexible voice belongs to the mother or good fairy. Just as children like extreme contrasts in movement lessons, so they like extreme contrasts in stories and poems, and these contrasts affect speech and movement alike.

Music as a stimulus

So much for miming fact and fiction; there remains music as the initial stimulus for mime. Play some exciting percussion music (perhaps very quick and strong) to dance to, then ask who or what would move in that way. The first character that the children suggest can be the beginning of a story created by the class. Contrast this with a piece of music, perhaps slow and light, to suggest another character and so build up a 'Noah's Ark' full of different people. The music need not always be percussion, but if you use recorded music, keep it short. Listening to music may give the children ideas for a mime. Music written as a description of animals might make a good beginning. Sometimes it may be wise to tell the children what the piece represents but not always as it may limit their ideas. A piece in which a composer meant to describe a hen might result in a child imitating a motor-car and this is all to the good. A final warning: titles of music may be given by the arranger or publisher as a selling gimmick and not by the composer.

CHAPTER IV

The Broadcast

The British Broadcasting Corporation presents a twenty-minute Music and Movement Programme on four mornings of the week during the school autumn, spring, and summer terms which is transmitted to Great Britain and Northern Ireland. There is one programme for the five- to six-year-old children and another for the six- to eight-year-olds. Both these programmes are repeated so that schools with many classes in each group can take the broadcasts. This repeat also gives broadcasters and producer an opportunity to follow the work done each week in a school.

The programmes are prepared in close co-operation with the schools. Since August 1959 children from a London school have attended the studio each week to take part in rehearsals and so help in the building of the programme. The script is also tried out, prior to broadcasting, on a class in a school in the Provinces; teachers from various Reporting Schools in the country and the BBC Education Officers report on response to the broadcast.

The budget for the programme allows for first-rate artists to take part. This, together with the wealth of music at hand in the music and gramophone libraries, offers a programme which is well worth considering as part of an Infant school timetable, even when a music specialist is available in the school. The planned schemes for the broadcast are approved by the Primary Committee of the School Broadcasting Council: the preparation of scripts is then carried out by the broadcaster and producer in charge of the series from the School Broadcasting Department.

Since the programme has to serve such a large variety of

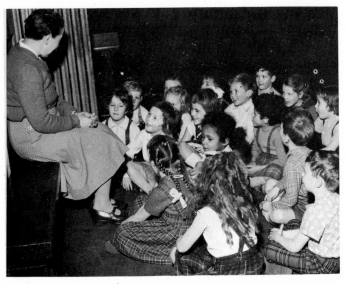

20   Listening

schools the overall scheme must be carefully planned. The whole content of the series must apply to the whole age group and yet offer sufficient progression. In the Music and Movement I series a specific element of music and movement—Time, Weight, or Space—forms a theme for each script. The stress throughout a programme could, for example, be on quick and slow. Towards the end of each programme the children are asked to gather round the wireless set for melody-making and listening. In the Music and Movement II series the programmes are based on the music and movement learnt in the first series, and dramatic themes are used.

In both series a certain amount of recapitulation is done at the beginning of each term to benefit the new entrants to classes, though it is better for a class to follow a whole year's course so that there is continuity and development. Repetition of movement is an essential part of the work so that children can develop individual styles through exploration of a single movement. Each repetition is accompanied by additional suggestions to help in this. Repetition of music is also important: a tune will become part of the children's musical repertoire through many hearings. It is surprising how many people recall their first memories of melodies through their experience of music and movement at the age of five.

The music chosen is always taken from the works of established composers. The snatches used are whole themes in themselves and give the children a store of worthwhile music. Orchestral records are very seldom used since it is easier for children to hear a single instrument than a full orchestra. The music is therefore arranged for instrumentalists who are chosen according to the content of the programme. A piccolo and bassoon could be chosen for contrasts of levels, a trombone and flute for contrasts of weight.

There is a teachers' leaflet which gives the aim of the series, and notes and suggestions for music to help those who use the broadcasts. At the end of every broadcast the music and movements are given at dictation speed to enable the teacher to take down details of music used. If this is missed it can be obtained by inquiry to the School Broadcasting Council.

The Studio. How the programmes are put together

Scripts and music, having been prepared previously, are brought to the studio. Broadcaster, instrumentalists, and producer then spend the first hour of rehearsal time trying out the music and fitting it to the numerous cues in the script; and sometimes there are as many as fifty of these cues. This is a long and arduous task for the artists, as playing numerous fragments of large works is very different from playing in concerts, even though the same artists may be famous soloists or leaders of great orchestras. The short pieces of music never last longer than thirty seconds in duration. Sometimes a whole section will be required, while at other times only half of it will be needed. Generally, two or three pieces of music will have been previously selected for each movement, and it is in this preliminary rehearsal time that the final choice is usually made. Sometimes the decision is left until the children arrive for the lesson, so that their response to the pieces of music will be the deciding factor.

Since a great number of pieces are played and the order is not straightforward, the music is written out on manuscript paper. This again adds to the difficulties of the artist, as reading from a manuscript copy is far more difficult than from a printed copy. Yet this must be done for the smooth running of the programme. In one way it helps the artist as he has to follow the words of the broadcaster as well as find the music to play, and this would be an impossible task if the music stand was cluttered with numerous sheets of music.

While this is going on, the Studio Manager (who is responsible for the sound you hear) places the artists and sets up microphones to give the best possible sound. This is very important as the response of the children is dependent on the quality of sound they hear.

Children from a local school then arrive in the studio for

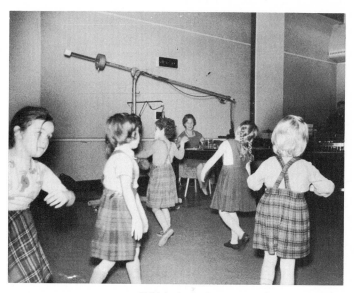

21 Children in the Studio

the first rehearsal. During this the programme is timed, and any difficulties which the children encounter in understanding commands or moving with the music are noted. Difficulties are ironed out by changing words, altering speeds of music, or even changing a piece of music entirely.

The final rehearsal which now follows should be an almost perfect performance, only the finest adjustments being made to timing. Because of the medium, additional pauses after each activity have to be made and 'key' words in the script have to be repeated. These rehearsals have taken over two hours and now all is ready for the final recording. At least six people, apart from the children and their teachers, have for several hours contributed to the production of a twenty-minute broadcast.

School Reception

A great many experiments have been made with different types of studios and microphone placing. In one school where the acoustics of the hall were very poor, it was found that loud-speakers hung in opposite corners of the hall, facing each other diagonally, gave good results. Previously there had only been one speaker and the teacher had been forced to repeat all commands.

To get the best out of the programmes it is essential for the radio set to be well tuned. It is better to set the volume control at half-way to maximum, and the speaker control to maximum. Any adjustment can then be made to volume control.

The part played by the teacher in the broadcasts must be an active one. The children should be helped verbally where necessary, but the teacher should never actually perform the movement, as the children will only copy and never interpret for themselves. Praise should always be given, especially if a generally poor child shows promise. Last of all, one should not be too ambitious for the children's response. If a child merely walks to slow music the mood has been captured, and that alone is sufficient at first. Progress is slow and children must be allowed to develop at their own rate.

CHAPTER V

Follow-up Lessons in Music

Besides following up the broadcast lessons by trying out again all the work covered in the programme, music and movement can be extended and developed in the classroom. This can be done in many ways.

Listening to Music

Music used for movement can be used again in the classroom for listening; the more familiar it is, the more the children will enjoy it. Programme music (a piece with a descriptive title), such as 'The Little Train of Caipira' by Villa Lobos or 'The Chicken on the Wall' by Inghelbrecht, could lead to the painting of a picture, clay modelling, free writing, the making of a frieze, the writing of a play, or poetry writing. Individual children might choose to do one of these or a small group might work together. Pieces without titles could still lead in the same direction, the children's imagination interpreting pictures the music paints for them.

The teacher should be ready to call attention to pieces which highlight one instrument. Pictures of instruments of the orchestra should already be at hand on the music table so that no opportunity is lost in linking the sound of the instrument with its appearance. There is no reason why the children should not become as familiar with the names of well-known composers, instruments or pieces as they are with, say, characters they see on the television. Large class books can form, either in pictures or words, a record of music made familiar through dancing and listening. Children might choose headings such as 'Our Trumpet Tunes', 'Bassoon Tunes', 'Strong Tunes', 'Gentle Tunes', 'Slow Tunes', or 'Quick Tunes' for these books. They will not be able to listen for long periods at a time. It is best to have short spells of listening, but the diet should be balanced as it is in a music and movement lesson. The children can become familiar with different tunes linked in a story as they are in *Peter and the Wolf* (Prokofiev) where the tunes and instruments used depict each character; or with tunes from a suite as in *The Carnival of Animals* (Saint-Saëns) where they are used to paint a series of musical pictures; with music contrasted in mood or music where instruments are featured. From the large class books children can be guided to choose music for class activities. They could select the incidental music for their own plays, for stories in mime, and for puppet plays.

Melody Making

Creating music can begin as early as any other Infant School activity. It can follow naturally from their play in the playground. Children call each other by name and in doing so often pitch notes at this interval:

This is a two-syllabled name and the stress is even—two even notes. The child has made a tune. Different names will give varied musical patterns.

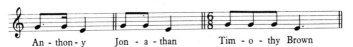

An - thon - y   Jon - a - than   Tim - o - thy Brown

Children can sing and tap these musical patterns and much
fun can be had between teacher and class with question and

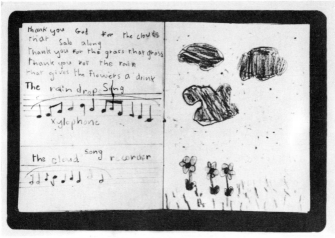

22   A page from Christine's own song book

answer patterns. This can be done in a very simple way at
first, the teacher singing somebody's name to 'lah' and the
children guessing and singing the name back. The common
words of the classroom can be included in this method of
melody making, and gradually whole sentences can be
built up such as:

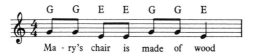

G   G   E   E   G   G   E
Ma - ry's chair   is   made   of   wood

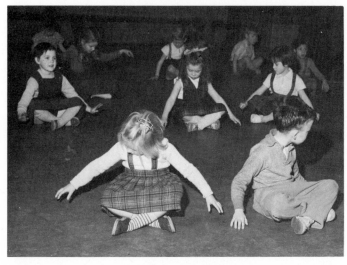

23   Tapping to music

The rhythm and tune can be given by the teacher, e.g.:

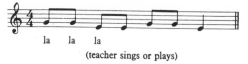

la   la   la

(teacher sings or plays)

and the words can be given by individual children. Then words and tune can be fitted together. The children can then be given merely a rhythm and can make up their own tune and words to fit it.

These examples use various rhythms but only two 'calling notes', G and E. These notes can form the basis of the easiest kind of scale that exists—the pentatonic scale—on which tunes such as 'Auld Lang Syne' and the verse of 'Will Ye No' Come Back Again?' are built. (In tonic sol-fa the notes are doh, ray, me, soh, and lah, and on the keyboard C, D, E, G, and A in the white-note scale.)

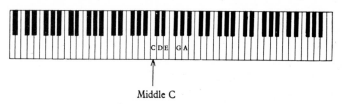

Middle C

As soon as the children have mastered two-note patterns, introduce a third note, lah—i.e. A in this case.

Here is an example from a child's repertoire:

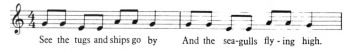

See the tugs and ships go by   And the sea-gulls fly-ing high.

The couplet was made up and the three-note tune added. Four- and five-note tunes can be built in the same way, adding first middle C: doh, then D: ray. When these five notes have been learned the major scale should present no difficulty to children.

All the work can be done without notation, but once a child has created a tune it would be very worth while to write it on a stave. Charts can be made for the children to follow. A group of children playing on percussion or melodic instruments could accompany the singers; in fact, the whole class can take part in the orchestration in some way or other. One group could have a counter rhythm which, at first, could be merely a regular pulse, so that the class were singing and playing in two parts. This work could be extended to playing in three, four, or as many parts as you have instruments.

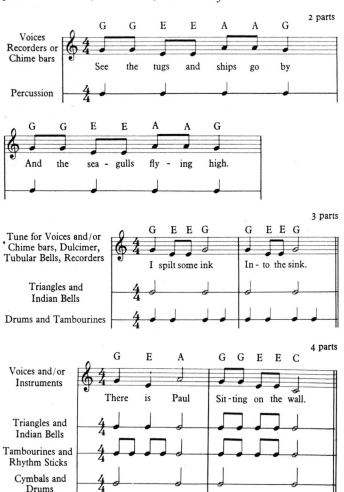

From simple beginnings such as these a great deal of valuable musical groundwork has been covered. The value lies

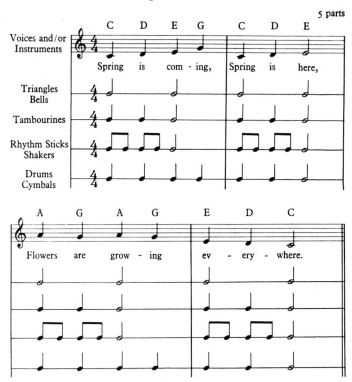

in the fact that the children have made music themselves. Melodic instruments such as chime bars, small xylophone, dulcimer, and tubular bells all have the names of the notes marked on them, so that the children could at first follow from a chart such as this with the notes named above:

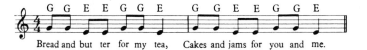

The children would become familiar with the placing of the notes and would soon be able to dispense with letters and

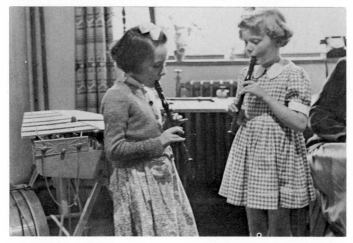

24   Playing a tune by ear, immediately after a singing lesson: 'My maid Mary'

read actual notation. This follows for tunes built of three, four, and five notes.

At the earliest stage of melody making, couplets made up round a theme could form the basis for a very short operetta. A narrator could relate the story and a group of singers and players could bring in the tune from time to time, either to introduce a character, add a comment, or even tell part of the tale. 'The Bremen Town-Musicians'[1] can be told like this, and 'The Gingerbread Man'[2] and 'The Tale of the Turnip'[3] also have repetitive choruses which work well.

Children need not always fit words to their tunes. They

[1] *Grimm's Fairy Tales* (Routledge and Kegan Paul, London).
[2] *Stories to Tell Children* by Sara Cone Bryant (Harrap).
[3] *Stories to Tell and How to Tell Them* by Elizabeth Clark (U.L.P.).

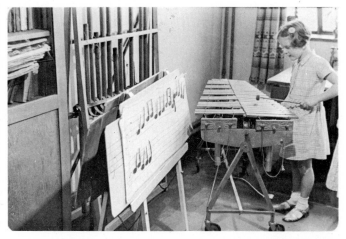

25 A seven-year-old playing her own tune from the flannel graph

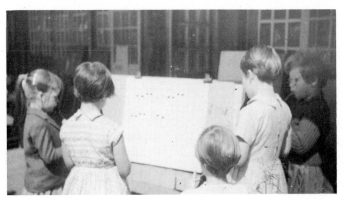

26 Recorders at playtime

could choose titles of movements used in music and movement lessons—*A Strong Tune, A Gentle Tune*—and suggest different percussive effects which would make their tune into a strong tune or a gentle tune. If children are allowed to use percussion in the music and movement lesson this work will lead on naturally. They can also experiment with all sorts of sound effects to depict characters, episodes and moods.

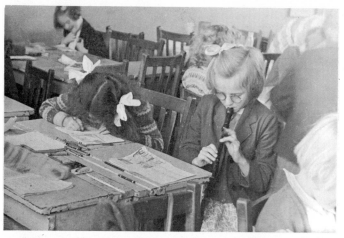

27 Seven-year-olds writing down original songs in their song books; a spontaneous activity taking place while others are painting, modelling, reading, etc.

These sound effects can be made without musical instruments: the children should be encouraged to experiment, as has been done recently in some dramatic productions, in making sounds with different surfaces and objects.

Experimenting with kitchen utensils would make a good beginning. Hitting different surfaces such as pots and pans, china mugs, or stone hot-water bottles with a wooden or metal spoon will give a variety of sounds. Additional noises

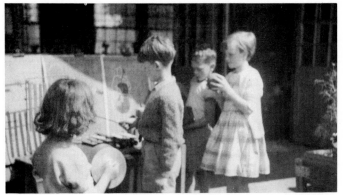

28 Making music with coconuts, drum, cymbals, and chime bars

can be made by blowing across the mouth of the hot-water bottle or a vacuum cleaner pipe, or by shaking paper, silk, leaves, or zinc sheeting. The pouring of liquids, foodstuffs— e.g. rice or sugar—or sand and gravel, and the movement of the hands or feet in or on these commodities, will give exciting sounds for incidental effects for the children's own plays and poetry.

The Making of Instruments

Linked with the making of sounds is the actual making of musical instruments themselves. One or two children in a class of six-year-olds in a Chiswick school made a complete set of drums from different-sized cake tins. Sheet rubber stretched across the open top, and sewn to the other side with string, kept the rubber taut: though they were crude, the drums made pleasant sounds and could be used in music making. Other children had partly filled cylinders with rice, sealing the top to keep the contents in and so making home-made maracas. The teacher herself was in the process of making a xylophone. (As the wood had to be

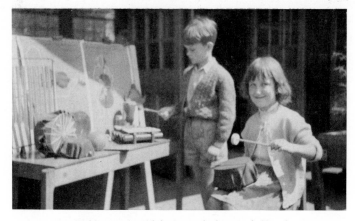

29   Making music with home-made drum and chime bars

cut to exact fractional measurements for the correct pitch of the notes the children could not undertake the making of this instrument themselves.) One boy had sand-papered strips of wood and was colouring them to make them look gay: he would then hit them together as rhythm sticks. What this one school could do, others could follow and even extend their range of instruments. Old 'cello and violin strings are very useful for making one-stringed fiddles, with the catgut stretched over a piece of wood attached to nails at either end. A piece of wood fixed three-quarters of the way up will act as a bridge so that different notes can be played. These instruments can supplement the percussion band, and all this creative work can be part of the normal activity period when the class are busy with their different interests. Instruments that the children make should all be available on the music table so that they are easily accessible when needed and can be experimented with.[1]

[1] See Kathleen M. Blocksidge, *Making Musical Apparatus and Instruments* (U.L.P.).

Recognizing Tunes

Listening and moving to music will give children a store of tunes to remember. The recognition of tunes can be helped by sequences in the music and movement lesson, where children show recognition of a melody by their different movements. This can lead, in their own creative music-making, to building tunes in certain patterns:

1. Tune A: Tune B
2. Tune A: Tune B: Tune A
3. Tune A: Tune B: Tune A: Tune C: Tune A.

These formulae can be found in most composed music. One child need not be the composer of the whole melody. Tony can supply Tune A, John Tune B, and so on. The children could them make up words suggesting movement and thus create their own dances.

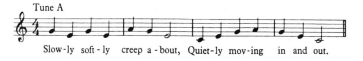

Tune A

Slow-ly soft-ly creep a-bout, Quiet-ly mov-ing in and out.

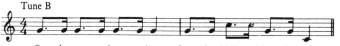

Tune B

On the spot we jump a-bout, jump-ing high and jump-ing low.

Music should permeate the whole Infant curriculum and should be a normal part of activities. There is no need for anyone to feel a stranger to it, as there are so many instruments, records, books, and broadcasts which can help the teacher.

CHAPTER VI

Follow-up Lessons in Movement

In going over the points made in the broadcast, a teacher can help enormously by interesting the shy, the clumsy, and the naughty as well as the children who respond well: tentative movements will become more confident if you encourage at the right time. Children working half-heartedly may need something harder to do such as:

'See if you can bend backwards as well as forwards.'
'Try lifting up your arms as well as a leg, very slowly, without wobbling over.'

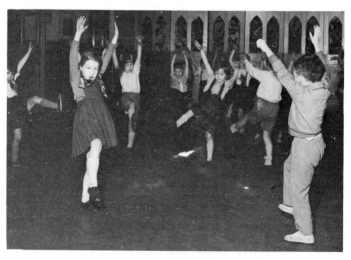

30 Lifting arms and legs slowly

There is much more opportunity to encourage individual development in a follow-up lesson than during the broadcast. (After all, no broadcaster can see your children.) No matter how slight this development may be, you must provide the next stage and also decide whether the rest of the class can benefit by it.

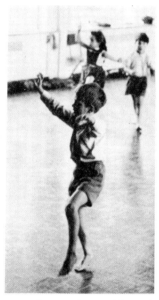

31 Boys can be graceful too!

'Johnnie drew a small circle with his finger; now, Johnnie, see if you can draw a circle with your elbow or foot.'

'Who can find a new way of drawing a circle?'

'Where can you draw a circle?'

'Find another place to draw a circle.'

Repetition often forms the whole of a follow-up, because children enjoy repeating a familiar movement. There is a danger, however, that too much repetition will produce slapdash movements: at the first sign of this, change the movement by stressing another element or direction.

Time
   'Curl and twist your whole body *slowly*.'
   'Curl and twist your whole body *quickly*.'
   'Make yourself as straight as you can, *quickly*.'
   'Very *slowly*, stretch out straight in a different way.'

Space
   'Find a space, quickly.'
   'Find a space *behind* you.'
   'Point to another space—now, jump *low down* near the floor to that space.'
   'Very slowly turn *round and round* in your space.'

Weight
   'Walk all over the floor.'
   'Walk as *heavily* as you can.'
   'Walk as *lightly* as you can.'

It may be possible with your own class to develop single movements into some sequence not used in the broadcast. This will teach co-ordination, flow of movement, and a feeling for phrasing. To feel a phrase is much more important at this stage than to be able to tap out three beats in a bar. Here is an example beginning with a single movement.

'Slowly grow up as tall as you can:
Slowly curl up on the floor as small as you can:
Now grow up tall and curl up small—very slowly:
See if you can grow up high and sink down low, as you
    dance round the room:
This time, slowly turn round and round as you dance up
    and down.'

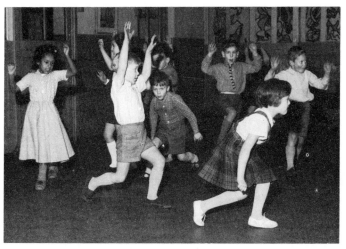

32   Dancing up and down

Use imagery sparingly at this stage. When you suggest
an image, you are really asking the children to extract its
movement qualities and this raises one more barrier. A
musical sound or the actual movement word will produce
immediate action. Later, when children have learned how to
move, imagery can be useful, as long as they really know
what you are talking about. Children ought to have some

experience of the image before they can be expected to interpret it.

Towards the end of the first year in Movement education children may be ready to dance with a partner. It may look as if they are dancing at the same time as, rather than *with*, a partner but this can be counteracted:

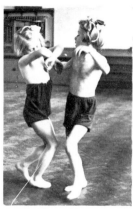

33   Dancing with a partner: Margaret and Lorraine in perfect harmony

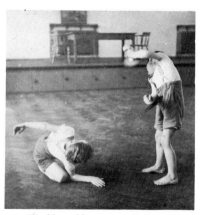

34   Working with a partner: Roger using cymbals and Keith moving accordingly

'Move slowly towards your partner and keep looking at her all the time.'

'You follow your partner: if she dances quickly, you dance quickly; if she dances slowly, you dance slowly.'

Moving in the opposite direction to a partner is exciting; one child can reach up high, while the other sinks down low. This can lead on to questions and answers in movement where the children can show in their movements whether they agree or disagree with each other. One child can move and the other answer back in movement. Two instruments, perhaps a tambour and tambourine, can help to keep a firm rein on the questions and answers.

Waiting for the other to move gives the child a time to watch and a time to dance. The teacher, too, must play a waiting game, because a long-term policy is just as important when you teach movement as it is when you teach reading and writing. Children must be given time to learn *how* to move, time to play percussion instruments, time to listen to music, and time to watch other children. Their rate of development may be slow, but once they have evolved their own individual style of movement it will remain with them whether they are playing games, dancing, or miming. You may have a future dancer, actress, or Olympic star in your class: your responsibility is great. Adult movements imposed on a child may appear to get quicker results but will look as artificial as powder and lipstick on a five-year-old.

Three questions must be answered in planning a movement lesson.

    1. 'What part of the body moves?'
    2. 'How does it move?'
    3. 'Where does it move?'

The large number of possible answers which have been suggested in Chapter I will give you a three-fold plan for a series of lessons. Each lesson must have a beginning, a middle, and an end!

The Beginning
 'Something old—something new' is as good a maxim as

any: begin with some familiar movements such as *running* or *stretching out in different directions*, and then add the new possibilities:

1. 'Run forwards, back, sideways, round and round, in and out, without bumping.'

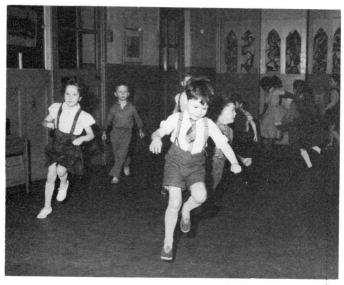

35   Making an energetic start

2. 'Run high up in the air, or low down near the floor.'
3. 'Run as fast as you can and stop quite still wherever you are when the drum stops.'
4. 'Run all over the floor, and when you hear the drum twist yourself into a knot and stay there.'

If space is too limited for vigorous running in all directions, it may make a better beginning to the lesson to stretch from narrow to wide.

1. 'Slowly stretch out wide—wider.'
2. 'Make yourself as thin as you can—quickly.'
3. 'Stretch out as wide as you can—quickly.'
4. 'Slowly shrink so that you are very thin and narrow.'
5. 'Stretch out as straight as you can—quickly.'
6. 'Curl and twist yourself into a knot—slowly.'

Very young and rather timid children need a different beginning. Gather them into a close group round you. Then, with a percussion instrument or your voice, send the children a little way away and bring them back to you again. Repeat this several times with as few words as you can. Now add something new—the children could move away low down on the floor and return high up in the air and vice versa. They could stride away from you and tiptoe back, perhaps backwards or sideways. There are infinite variations if you remember to work on the principle of contrast, that is from quick to slow, strong to light, straight to twisted, high to low.

If the hall is not big enough for this simple activity, the children can move upwards instead of outwards. Reaching up to the ceiling and sinking down to the floor has many variations, and the deliberate use of the floor gives the children the feeling of security they may need.

Various parts of the body can lead this movement: chest, knee, foot, chin, back, as well as the hands. A choice such as 'elbow or big toe' will give the children a chance to decide for themselves which part shall lead the movement, and an opportunity to develop their originality.

The beginning of a lesson will depend on the mood of your class. Moving on the spot (reaching up to the ceiling or stretching out wide), may be more sensible than running in different directions, but if the children are in an energetic mood, fast running with sudden stops will use up their surplus energy and give you the discipline you want.

The Middle

You will have decided on the theme you wish to emphasize; it may be Time, Space, or Weight, and although none of these can be isolated in any movement, Time—quick and slow—is perhaps the easiest to begin with.

Time

If you consider *what* parts of the body can move quickly and slowly, *how* and *where* they can move, this will provide you with ample material for the middle of your lessons.

1. 'Shake your head quickly.'
2. 'Shake your shoulders quickly.'
   'Shake your head, hands, and feet.'
   'Shake your whole body, shake all over.'
   'Shake high up in the air and low down on the floor, shake up and down all over the room.'
3. 'Walk as slowly as you can.'
4. 'Turn round as you walk, slowly.'
5. 'Try to touch the floor and ceiling as you walk slowly round and round.'

Space

In another lesson Space might well be your primary concern. Suggestions such as:

1. 'Find a space for yourself quickly.'
2. 'Look around until you see a space—now jump into it.'
3. 'Walk on your heels to another space behind you.'
4. 'Slowly turn round and round in your space.'

will give experience in finding a space in the hall. Now they are in a space, particular uses of it can be taught.

1. 'Move your arms all round you; feel the air above your head, low down, behind you, at the side of you, in front of you.'
2. 'Stretch out wide.'
3. 'Curl up as small as you can.'
4. 'Draw a circle on the floor.'
5. 'Tiptoe round in your circle.'
6. 'Jump round in your circle.'
7. 'Jump low down near the floor in your own circle.'
8. 'Draw a circle above your head or at the side of you.'
9. 'Draw a circle right round yourself with your head or elbow or foot.'
10. 'Now draw circles everywhere—make up a "circle dance".'

Weight

Another lesson could be based on strong and light movements. Imaginative use of percussion will explain the difference between strong and light. This accompaniment can be played on one instrument such as the tambour, or on two instruments, say the triangle and tambour.

1. 'Press your feet into the floor—press down.
   Walk slowly and heavily pressing your feet down into the floor.'—*Tambour* (slow).

2. 'Make your feet dance quickly all over the floor without making a noise. Hardly touch the floor.'— *Triangle* (quick).

3. 'Punch and kick with your arms and legs as hard as you can.'— *Tambour* (quick).

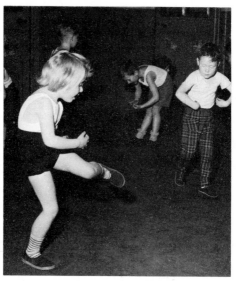

36   Curling and twisting dance

4. 'Lift your arms up very slowly and lightly—lift right up to the ceiling.'— *Triangle* (slow).

5. 'Lift your arms and one leg up as high as you can—very slowly and lightly.'— *Triangle* (slow).

6. 'Now move gently round the room, lifting your arms and legs high up in the air before you step.'— *Triangle* (slow).

The End

A movement lesson should lead into a dance of some kind or group work; although Infants are too young to have any real group feeling, they can enjoy moving together in small groups.

Group work can easily be introduced with percussion in-

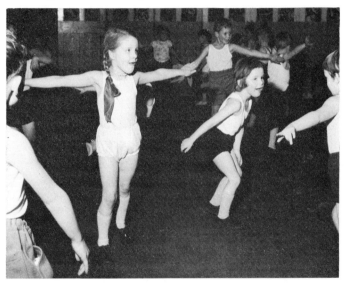

37   Straight dance

struments. The class can be divided into small groups, each following an instrument played by one child in each group. This 'follow-my-leader' is simple and enjoyable, especially if the leader is encouraged to alter the time, weight, and direction. Such instruments as castanets, tambourines, and tambours give many different movement qualities yet do not stop the player from moving.

Just as an actor decides when to raise his voice, when to whisper, when to take the stage, and when to withdraw, so must a teacher. There will be times in the lesson when a whisper will command deep attention; at other times a louder voice will stimulate greater activity. Teachers must

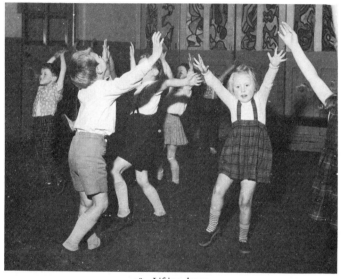

38   Lifting dance

sense when to take a back seat and give the children time to experiment themselves. *They must never demonstrate the actual movement* but indicate the idea of the movement in their voice and accompaniment.

Don't talk too much, and never at the same time as percussion or music. If you speak and play at the same time, you are asking the children to do *three* things at once: to listen to what you are saying; to listen to the music; and to move. Pauses between speech and music should vary according to the movement. If the movement is quick you can end your speech with 'quickly' and play immediately, but if the movement is to be slow, a longer pause between speech and music will give the idea of 'slowly' much better.

A plan of a lesson should be adjusted immediately if the children need more repetition or if they invent some interesting movement which can be developed further so that the rest of the class can benefit by it. When you ask children to demonstrate their own movements, always choose two or three different interpretations, so that the class realize there are many ways of moving.

In Appendix A there are some suggestions for lessons based on Time, Weight, and Space. The balance of the lessons will be left to you as repetition and development will depend on each class. Music, percussion, or the voice can be used in teaching the following movement lessons.

Percussion or the voice may also be used as a signal to stop. In this way the children will have a chance to move in their own time without music, until they are stopped by some pre-arranged signal.

'When you hear the drum stop wherever you are.'

These lessons can be developed in many ways by emphasizing different qualities and directions. The children will show in their own movements where they need more help. To suggest here the further needs of *your* children would be futile, but perhaps these lessons will serve as a 'starting-off' point.

There are no set movements to be learnt by a certain age group; beginners of any age will have to master moving in time with strong and light qualities and with some shape and form to their movements. There are many ways of teaching movement to older age groups. You can use a dramatic angle, visual stimuli such as patterns or pictures, everyday working actions, poetry . . . and music. Five-year-olds have a limited experience, vocabulary, and co-ordination of movement. Approach through music—even if it is only percussion—is the simplest and most direct method of overcoming these limitations. Once over them, the whole world of dance lies beyond.

Movement is for everybody, of whatever age, whether they are performers or merely onlookers. To appreciate the pattern of cricket, rugger, and football, the subtle movements of an actor as well as the beauty and excitement of the many dance forms, is the reward of an education in Music and Movement.

Appendix A

SUGGESTIONS FOR LESSONS
BASED ON TIME, WEIGHT, AND SPACE

TIME

1. 'Dance quickly and when the music stops, you stop—quite still.'
2. 'The music will keep stopping—you dance quickly and then stop every time the music stops.'
3. 'Spin round quickly in a space by yourself.'
4. 'Curl up on the floor as small as you can—quickly.'
5. 'Very slowly grow up as tall as you can.'
6. 'Curl up again quickly.'
7. 'This time, let your side or elbow or chin go up to the ceiling first—slowly up.'
8. 'Curl up again quickly.'
9. 'Now, move up to the ceiling slowly and curl up again quickly.'
10. 'Keep moving up to the ceiling slowly and curling up again quickly.'
11. 'Up to the ceiling quickly.'
12. 'Curl up again quickly.'
13. 'Now see if you can dance up to the ceiling and down to the floor quickly; up and down—quickly.'
14. 'Do that very slowly; slowly dance up and down.'
15. 'This time turn round and round as you dance up and down slowly.'
16. 'Stand still: Look at the ceiling.'
17. 'Nod your head at the ceiling quickly.'

18. 'Move your hands up to the ceiling quickly.'
19. 'Move one foot up to the ceiling quickly.'
20. 'Let your head, hands and feet dance right up to the ceiling.'
21. 'Dance up to the ceiling as quickly as you can.'
22. 'Look at the floor: slowly walk low down near the floor, on your feet or on your hands and feet.'

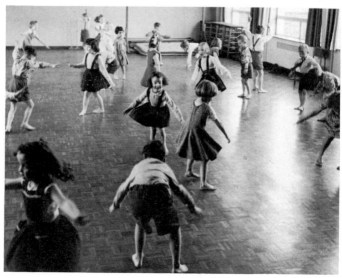

39   Spinning round quickly

23. 'Find another way of moving slowly, low down near the floor.'
24. 'See if you can turn round slowly as you move low down near the floor.'
25. 'Now dance as quickly as you can high up in the air. Then dance low down near the floor slowly.'
26. 'Stand still: tap on the floor with your toes quickly.'

27. 'Tap on the floor with your heels.'
28. 'Now make up a heel and toe dance: dance forwards, backwards, sideways, and round and round.'
29. 'Your heel and toe dance was very quick; see if you can clap or nod or sway very slowly to this music.'
30. 'This time the music will start slowly then get faster and faster and end with a bang; you follow the music carefully —clap slowly, then faster and faster. '
31. 'Now see if you can dance slowly, then faster and faster.'
32. 'Dance with your whole body, first slowly, then faster and faster.'
33. 'This time, the music will end differently; see if you can follow it straight away. Dance up and down and round and round.'
34. 'The music was slow then fast then slow again; you dance to it again—dance all over the floor, slowly, then quickly, then again slowly.'
35. 'Very slowly tiptoe out of the hall' (or 'to your clothes and get dressed', etc.)

WEIGHT

1. 'Stamp on the floor; stamp forwards, backwards, sideways, and round and round.'
2. 'Up on your toes, as lightly as you can, tiptoe in and out quickly; hardly touch the floor.'
3. 'Stamp; Tiptoe; Stamp; Tiptoe.'
4. 'Jump as high as you can.'
5. 'Jump backwards or sideways.'
6. 'Jump low down near the floor.'
7. 'Turn round as you jump.'
8. 'Stand still; very gently sway from side to side.'
9. 'Sway your head and shoulders; sway your whole body slowly and lightly.'

10. 'Now, kick out one leg as hard as you can; kick out behind you, at the side of you, or high up in the air.'
11. 'Clench your fists; make your arms strong.'
12. 'Punch down to the floor.'
13. 'Punch high up in the air.'
14. 'Punch all round you.'

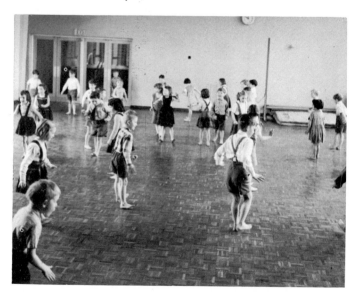

40   Walking on heels

15. 'Make up a strong kicking and punching dance.'
16. 'Very smoothly and lightly, glide one foot along the floor.'
17. 'Glide your other foot along the floor.'
18. 'Glide round the room very smoothly and gently.'
19. 'Now kick out your arms and legs as you jump in the air.'
20. 'Lift up one foot; press your foot into the floor very slowly and heavily.'

21. 'Lift up your other foot; press your foot into the floor very slowly and heavily.'
22. 'Walk as heavily as you can, pressing your feet into the floor slowly and heavily.'
23. 'Now dance *off* the floor as lightly as you can; make your feet dance high up in the air quickly and lightly.'
24. 'Curl up on the floor; very gently, lift up to the ceiling and stay there.'
25. 'Flop down to the floor heavily.'
26. 'Slowly lift up to the ceiling, lightly and gently; then flop down to the floor as heavily as you can.'
27. 'See if you can turn round as you lift up gently and flop down heavily all over the room.'
28. 'Glide along the floor very gently to me and sit down here without touching the floor with your hands.'
29. 'Clap your hands or slap the floor, quickly and loudly.'
30. 'Now tap as slowly and softly as you can.'
31. 'See if the boys can dance while the girls clap quickly and loudly: a quick, strong dance, boys.'
32. 'This time the boys will tap very quietly while the girls make up a slow light dance.'
33. 'Now, everybody dance: I will play quickly and loudly; then very quietly and slowly.'

SPACE

1. 'Run in and out of each other without bumping.'
2. 'Run quickly in a twisted line; make your feet dance in a twisted line, in and out.'
3. 'Walk in a straight line.'
4. 'Look behind you; walk backwards in a straight line.'
5. 'Walk sideways in a straight line.'
6. 'Twist in and out of each other quickly.'

7. 'Point to a space; walk on your heels in a straight line to your space.'
8. 'Curl up on the floor.'

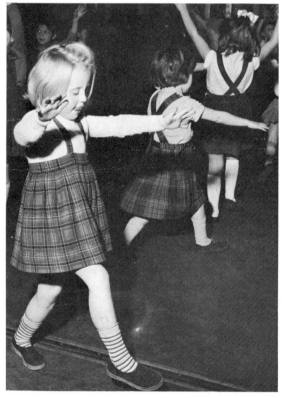

41   Walking in a straight line

9. 'Shoot out one leg as straight as you can.'
10. 'Curl up again.'
11. 'Shoot out one arm as straight as you can.'

12. 'Shoot out your head as straight as you can.'
13. 'Shoot out your arms, legs, and head as straight as you can.'
14. 'Stand up quickly; shoot out your arms and legs and head as straight as you can, all round you.'
15. 'Can you jump with straight arms and legs?'
16. 'Make up a lot of different straight jumps.'
17. 'Jump out as straight and as wide as you can.'
18. 'Very slowly curl and twist your hands, curl and twist your arms, your head, your shoulder, back, tummy, legs; curl and twist yourself up into a knot, slowly.'
19. 'Jump out as straight as you can.'
20. 'Very slowly, curl and twist yourself up into a knot.'
21. 'Very slowly grow out as straight as you can sideways or backwards.'
22. 'Very quickly, curl and twist yourself into a knot.'
23. 'Slowly grow out as straight as you can.'
24. 'Twist yourself into a knot quickly.'
25. 'You've made up a lot of straight jumps; see if you can make up a lot of twisted jumps; twist yourself into the air as you jump.'
26. 'Now make up a jumping dance: straight jumps and twisted jumps.'
27. 'Slowly, kneel down on the floor.'
28. 'Draw a big circle on the floor.'
29. 'Draw a circle above your head.'
30. 'Draw a circle at the side of you or behind you.'
31. 'Draw a small circle, then a bigger circle, then the biggest circle you can draw.'
32. 'Your biggest circle can go from one side of the room to the other; first draw your small circle, then a bigger circle, then a circle as big as you can make it.'
33. 'Now make up a circle dance—draw circles with your head, hands, knees, elbows and feet.'

Appendix B

MUSIC SUITABLE FOR MOVEMENT

A great deal of the listed music in this Appendix can be obtained as gramophone recordings. Gramophone catalogues giving information of the current recordings of works can be obtained from any music shop or record shop. The public libraries also are always willing to give this sort of information.

1. PIANO COMPOSITIONS
AND PIANO ARRANGEMENTS

The asterisk denotes music that is fairly easy to play. Most pieces have the melody in the right hand and it is far better to play musically and up to time with one hand than stumble through a piece using both hands. The melody line can be played on any melodic instrument.

The amount of music selected should be very short, probably the first eight or sixteen bars. For strong movements twenty seconds of music should be the limit; for light movements thirty seconds. A list of publishers' addresses may be found on pages 109 and 110.

Quick light movements		*Publishers*
Bach	French Suites:	Augener
	★Suite III, Minuet 1	
	Suite IV, Gigue	
	Suite V, Gavotte	
	Suite VI, Bourrée	
	Notebook of Anna Magdalena Bach:	
	★Musette in D	Boosey and Hawkes

Barber	Souvenirs—Ballet Suite, Op. 28	Schirmer
	Two Step	
	Schottische	
Bartók	*For Children:	Boosey and Hawkes
	Vol. I, Nos. 1, 4, 8, 10, 15, 23, 27, 29	
	Vol II, Nos. 3, 6, 18, 20, 30	
Bizet	Jeux d'Enfants:	Durand
	Les Chevaux de Bois	
	Les Bulles de Savon	
	Le Bal	
	L'Arlésienne Suite:	
	*Farandole	
Brahms	Waltzes, Op. 39, Nos. 6, 10	Augener
Delibes	Sylvia:	Heugel
	Dance of the Ethiopians	
Dvořák	Slavonic Dances, Op. 46:	Lengnick
	Nos. 1, 3, 5, 6, 7, 8	
Grieg	Holberg Suite: Op. 40, No. 5	Peters
	Rigaudon	
	Peer Gynt Suite:	
	Arabian Dance	
Haydn	String Quartet, Op. 54, No. 3	Boosey and
	*Allegro (arr. Yvonne Adair)	Hawkes
	*Two Little Dances (arr. Yvonne Adair)	
		Boosey and Hawkes
Mussorgsky	Pictures from an Exhibition:	Augener
	Ballet of Unhatched Chicks	
	Limoges. Le Marché	
	4th Promenade	
Ravel	Le Tombeau de Couperin:	Durand
	Toccata	
Rossini arr. Respighi		Chester
	La Boutique Fantasque:	
	Can-Can	

Schumann	★Album for the Young:	Augener
	Nos. 3, 5, 11, 14	
	Papillons:	Augener
	Nos. 4, 9	
	Carnaval:	
	Papillons	
	Lettres Dansantes	
	Pantalon et Colombine	
Shostakovich	Golden Age Ballet: International Music Co.	
	Polka	
Tchaikovsky	★Album for the Young:	Augener
	Nos. 2, 5, 8, 13, 14, 17	
	The Sleeping Beauty:	Paxton
	Red Riding Hood	
	Nutcracker Suite:	Rahter
	Dance of the Reed Pipes	
Walton	★Music for Children:	O.U.P.
	Nos. 1, 2, 4, 6, 9	
	Façade:	O.U.P.
	First Suite: Polka	
	Tango Pasadoblé	
	(middle section)	
	Tarantella	
	Second Suite: Scotch Rhapsody	
	Country Dance	
	Popular Song	
Warlock	Capriol Suite:	Curwen
	Tordion	
	Bransles	

★Nursery Rhymes (Oxford Nursery Song Book)   O.U.P.
    A Frog he would a-wooing go
    Girls and boys come out to play
    Hey diddle diddle
    Dance to your daddy

Here we go round the mulberry bush
Lucy Locket
Little boy blue
Little Jack Horner
Little Polly Flinders
The man in the moon
The Miller of Dee
Nuts in May
Polly put the kettle on
Simple Simon
The spider and the fly

Quick and Strong Movements

Bartók	★For Children:	Boosey and Hawkes
	Vol. I, Nos. 12, 33, 37, 40	
	Vol. II, Nos. 1, 3 (last part),	
	5 (var. 3), 8, 13, 21, 22, 27,	
	29, 31, 36 (differing rhythms)	
	Allegro Barbaro	Universal Edition
Bizet	Jeux d'Enfants:	Durand
	La Toupie	
	Trompette et Tambour	
Brahms	Handel Variations:	Augener
	Var. 1, 4, 7, 10, 15, 23	
	Waltzes, Op. 39:	
	Nos. 1, 4	
Delibes	Coppélia:	Fürstner
	Mazurka	
Dvořák	Slavonic Dances, Op. 46:	Lengnick
	Nos. 1, 2, 3, 5, 6, 7, 8	
Holst	The Planets: (2 piano version	Curwen
	Jupiter adaptable)	
	Mars	
	Uranus	

Howells	Lambert's Clavichord: Hughes's Ballet	O.U.P.
Mussorgsky	Pictures from an Exhibition: 1st and 5th Promenade Baba-Yaga	Augener
	Gopak	Augener
Rossini, arr. Respighi		
	La Boutique Fantasque: Tarantella *Cosaque	Chester
Schumann	*Album for the Young: Nos. 2, 7, 8, 12, 23, 29, 31, 36 Papillons: No. 3 Carnaval: Coquette Marche des Davidsbündler	Augener
Strauss	Der Rosenkavalier: Waltz	Chappell
Stravinsky	Le Baiser de la Fée: Peasant Dance	Boosey and Hawkes
Tchaikovsky	*Album for the Young: No. 3	Augener
Walton	*Music for Children: No. 7	O.U.P.
Warlock	Capriol Suite: *Basse Danse Bransles *Mattachins	Curwen
*Nursery Rhymes (Oxford Nursery Song Book) Polichinelle Pop goes the weasel Ride a cock horse Taffy was a Welshman		O.U.P.

Alternations of Quick and Light and Quick and Strong Movements

| Bach | Notebook of Anna Magdalena Bach: |

	*Polonaise in F (arr. Y. Adair)	
		Boosey and Hawkes
Bartók	*For Children:	Boosey and Hawkes
	Vol. I, Nos. 6, 19, 20, 21, 30	
	(high and low; light and strong);	
	38 (gradual crescendo to quick,	
	strong). Vol. II, No. 14 (changes	
	of pitch)	
Bizet	L'Arlésienne Suite:	Choudens
	*Farandole	
	Intermezzo (Minuetto)	
	Jeux d'Enfants:	Durand
	Les Chevaux de Bois	
Dvcřák	Slavonic Dances, Op. 46:	Lengnick
	Nos. 1, 3, 5, 6, 7, 8	
Haydn	Symphony No. 86 in D	Boosey and Hawkes
	*Minuetto (arr. Y. Adair)	
Holst	The Planets:	Curwen
	Uranus	
Martini	*Gavotte (arr. Y. Adair)	Boosey and Hawkes
Mouret	*Bourrée (arr. Y. Adair)	Boosey and Hawkes
Schubert	*Peasant's Dance (arr. Y. Adair)	
		Boosey and Hawkes
Schumann	Papillons: Nos. 6, 8	Augener
Warlock	Capriol Suite:	Curwen
	Bransles	
*Nursery Rhyme (Oxford Nursery Song Book)		O.U.P.
Hot cross buns		

Slow and Light Movements

Bach	*Minuet in G (arr. Y. Adair)	
		Boosey and Hawkes
Barber	Souvenirs––Ballet Suite:	Schirmer
	Waltz and Pas de Deux	

Bartók	*For Children:	Boosey and Hawkes

Bartók   ★For Children: Boosey and Hawkes
          Vol. I, Nos. 2, 3, 7, 11, 13, 17, 22, 24, 31
          ★Vol. II, No. 5 (Variations 1 and 2)
             Nos. 7, 9, 10, 11 (last half), 12, 16,
                24, 25, 28, 33, 34

Beethoven   Romance from Sonatina in G
              (arr. Y. Adair)   Boosey and Hawkes
          Bagatelle in F, Op. 33, No. 3
              (arr. Y. Adair)

Bizet   Jeux d'Enfants: Durand
          La Poupée

Brahms   Waltzes, Op. 39:   Augener
          Nos. 2, 3★, 7, 8, 9★, 15★
          Waltzes, Op. 52, Liebeslieder (duet
             version adaptable): Nos. 6, 10
          Handel Variations:
             Var. 2, 6, 11, 22
          Paganini Variations: Var. VI   Schirmer

Delibes   Coppélia: Fürstner
          ★Waltz from Act I

Delius   Hassan Serenade   Boosey and Hawkes

Dvořák   ★Waltz, Op. 54, No. 1   Simrock
          Slavonic Dances, Op. 46:   Lengnick
             Nos. 2, 4

Grieg   Peer Gynt Suite: Peters
          Morning
          Norwegian Melodies, Op. 17:
          ★Cowkeeper's Tune

Holst   The Planets: Curwen
          Saturn
          Venus

Jaubert   Valse Grise ('Un Carnet de Bal')
                   Macmelodies Ltd.

Mussorgsky	Pictures from an Exhibition:	Augener
	Il Vecchio Castello	
	2nd Promenade	
Ravel	Pièce en forme de Habanera	Leduc
	Mother Goose:	Durand
	Pavane	
	Valses Nobles et Sentimentales, No. 3	

Rossini–Respighi

	La Boutique Fantasque:	Chester
	Valse	
Schumann	Carnaval:	Augener
	Eusebius	
	Chopin	
	Nachtstück, Op. 23, No. 4	
Strauss	★Emperor's Waltz	Cranz
Tchaikovsky	★Album for the Young:	Augener
	Nos. 6, 7, 21	
Walton	★Music for Children:	O.U.P.
	Nos. 3, 5, 8	
	Façade:	
	First Suite: Valse	
	Tango	
	Swiss Yodelling Song	
	Second Suite: Noche Espagnole	
Warlock	Capriol Suite:	Curwen
	★Pieds en l'Air	

★Nursery Rhymes (Oxford Nursery Song Book)		O.U.P.
	Au clair de la lune	
	Bye Baby Bunting	
	I love little pussy	
	Curly Locks	
	Ladybird	
	Lavender's Blue	
	Little Bo-peep	

The north wind doth blow
Pat a cake
Pussy cat, Pussy cat, where have you been?
See-saw, Margery Daw
There was a lady loved a swine
How does my lady's garden grow?
Hush a bye, baby

Slow and Strong Movements

Albeniz	Tango, Op. 165, No. 2	Schott
Bartók	*For Children:	Boosey and Hawkes
	Vol. I, No. 18	
	Vol. II, 2, 11, 15, 32, 38	
Brahms	Handel Variations, Var. 9	Augener
Delibes	Sylvia:	Heugel
	*Prelude (opening)	
	Coppélia:	Fürstner
	*Czardas	
Dvořák	Slavonic Dances, Op. 46, No. 4	Lengnick
Falla	Ritual Fire Dance	Chester
Grieg	Sigurd Jorsalfar (Prelude)	Peters
Holst	The Planets:	Curwen
	Jupiter (middle section)	
	Saturn	
Mussorgsky	Pictures from an Exhibition:	Augener
	3rd Promenade	
	Part of Gnomus (descending octaves)	
Warlock	Capriol Suite:	Curwen
	*Pavane	
*Nursery Rhymes (Oxford Nursery Song Book)		O.U.P.
	London's Burning	
	Hark, hark, the dogs do bark	
	Upon Paul's Steeple	

Alternations of Slow and Light and Slow and Strong *(the changes are either gradual or sudden)*

Bartók	*For Children:	Boosey and Hawkes
	Vol. I, No. 16	
Dvořák	Slavonic Dances, Op. 46, No. 4	Lengnick
Grieg	*The Death of Åse (Peer Gynt)	Peters
Holst	The Planets:	Curwen
	Saturn	
Mussorgsky	Pictures from an Exhibition:	Augener
	Bydlo	
Schubert	*German Dance, Op. 33, No. 7	
	(arr. Y. Adair)	Boosey and Hawkes
Walton	*Music for Children, No. 10	O.U.P.

Alternations from Quick and Strong to Slow and Light

Bartók	*For Children:	Boosey and Hawkes
	Vol. I, Nos. 5, 14, 39	
Brahms	Hungarian Dance, No. 6	Lengnick
Dvořák	Slavonic Dances, Op. 46, No. 2	Lengnick

Alternations from Quick and Light to Slow and Strong

Bartók	*For Children:	Boosey and Hawkes
	Vol. II, No. 14	
Brahms	Hungarian Dance, No. 5	Lengnick
	(vivace section)	

Alternations from Slow and Light to Quick and Light

Bartók	*For Children:	Boosey and Hawkes
	Vol. II, No. 9	
Liszt	Hungarian Rhapsody, No. 2	Augener
Schumann	*Album for the Young, No. 9	Augener
Walton	Façade:	O.U.P.
	First Suite: Tango	

Alternations from Slow and Strong to Quick and Strong

Brahms	Hungarian Dance, No. 5	Lengnick
	(allegro section)	
Holst	The Planets:	Curwen
	Jupiter (middle section)	

More examples for changes from slow to quick and vice versa, together with other qualities are to be found in the Hungarian Dances of Brahms and Liszt, the Slavonic Dances of Dvořák, and much of Chopin's piano music.

2. EXAMPLES OF MUSIC AND PERCUSSION EFFECTS FOR SPECIFIC MOVEMENTS

LOCOMOTION

Running

(*a*) Bartók: For Children. Vol I, No. 29.

(*b*) Yankee Doodle.

Quick, even, regular beats tapped with the fingers or with a padded stick on a drum or tambour. Hard sticks used on a wooden block or temple blocks, or castanets.

Walking

(*a*) Mussorgsky: The Promenades from Pictures from an Exhibition.

(*b*) Frère Jacques.

As for running though the beat will be slower.

Leaping

(*a*) Bizet: Les Chevaux de Bois from Jeux d'Enfants.

(*b*) The Keel Row.

Leaping rhythm played on drum or tambour with a hard stick. Tambourines struck with the palm of the hand.

Striding

(*a*) Delibes: Prelude from Sylvia.

(*b*) Ding, Dong, Bell.

Gong or cymbal hit with a padded stick at regular intervals or cymbals clashed together keeping a regular beat.

Hopping and Jumping

(*a*) Bizet: Trompette et Tambourin from Jeux d'Enfants.

(*b*) Pop goes the Weasel.

Temple block or wooden block hit with hard sticks or rhythm sticks, using jumping rhythm.

Galloping

(*a*) Schumann: The Wild Horseman from Album for the Young (No. 8).

(*b*) Ride a Cock Horse.

As for jumping but use a galloping rhythm. A good effect can also be obtained by hitting together the rims of two half coconut shells in a galloping rhythm.

Walking on Hands and Feet

(*a*) Warlock: Pavane from Capriol Suite.

(*b*) One, two, buckle my shoe.

Gong, cymbal or drum hit softly with padded stick.

Creeping

(*a*) Schumann: Nachtstück, Op. 23, No. 4.

(*b*) Little Bo-peep.

Chime bars, or Indian bells tapped together at regular intervals; or drum or tambour hit with fingertips or wire brush; or temple blocks hit with a rubber-headed stick.

Tiny Steps

(*a*) Rossini–Respighi: Can-Can from La Boutique Fantasque.

(*b*) Lucy Locket.
Castanets or rhythm sticks; or temple blocks or wooden block hit with hard sticks.

TIME

Clapping Dance
(*a*) Bartók: For Children, Vol. I, No. 21.
(*b*) Dame, get up and bake your pies.
Castanets played in a clapping, rhythmic pattern; or rhythm sticks or temple blocks or wooden block hit with hard sticks.

Tapping with Toes and Heels
(*a*) Bizet: Intermezzo (Minuetto) from L'Arlésienne.
(*b*) This Old Man.
Castanets, or rhythm sticks or temple blocks or wooden block hit with hard sticks. Play quick, regular, even beats.

Slow to quick Dance
(*a*) Brahms: Hungarian Dance, No. 5.
(*b*) Three blind mice.
Tambourine played slowly with finger-tips at first and then shaken or tapped quickly.

Slow-quick-slow Dance
(*a*) Dvořák: Slavonic Dance, Op. 46, No. 2.
As above but return to slow tapping to finish.

SPACE

Curling and Twisting
(*a*) Schumann: Eusebius from Carnaval.
(*b*) Curly Locks.
A tambourine shaken and hit softly with finger tips, or a cymbal hit with padded stick in a continuous roll, or wire brush drawn across a drum.

Straight Dance

(*a*) Bartók: For Children, Vol II, No. 29.

(*b*) The Keel Row.

Cymbals clashed together giving crisp clashes; or wooden block or drum hit with hard sticks.

Circle Dance

(*a*) Bartók: For Children, Vol. II, No. 9.

(*b*) Pussy Cat, Pussy Cat, Where have you been?

Gong or single cymbal hit softly with a padded stick; or chime bars or Indian bells played gently.

WEIGHT

Lifting Dance

(*a*) Rossini–Respighi: Valse from La Boutique Fantasque.

(*b*) The Man in the Moon.

Crescendo and diminuendo rolls made with a padded stick on a cymbal or a crescendo and diminuendo made by shaking a tambourine.

Kicking, Punching, Stamping

(*a*) Bartók: For Children, Vol. II, No. 31.

(*b*) Polichinelle.

Drum, tambour, or tambourine hit with a hard stick, or cymbals clashed together.

Sliding

(*a*) Strauss, J.: Emperor's Waltz.

(*b*) See Saw, Margery Daw.

Swaying

(*a*) Delius: Serenade from Hassan.

(*b*) Bye, Baby Bunting.

Swinging

(*a*) Strauss, R.: Waltz from Der Rosenkavalier.

(*b*) Oh! Dear! What can the matter be?

Chime bars and tubular bells can be used effectively for sliding, swaying and swinging. A waltz rhythm will help all three movements and a tune made up with the five notes (see Chapter V), using one note for each swing, sway or slide will give the music for the movement. Alternatively a gong hit with a padded stick will give continuity of sound which is needed for the flow of these movements.

3. RECORDS AND OTHER MUSIC USEFUL FOR MOVEMENT

Records

Listen, Move, and Dance. A set of records designed for movement

Records 1 and 2. Very short pieces from well-known works arranged and directed by Vera Gray   HMV 7 EG 8727–8

Record 3. Electronic Sound Patterns composed and created by Daphne Oram in collaboration with Vera Gray

HMV 7 EG 8762

Record 4. Side 1. Moving Percussion composed by Vera Gray. Side 2. Electronic Sound Pictures composed and created by Desmond Briscoe in collaboration with Vera Gray

HMV CLP 3531

Stories in Movement. Devised by Rachel Percival

1. Persephone. By Peter Wishart   HMV 7 EG 8976
2. Beowulf. By Peter Wishart   HMV 7 EG 8977
3. Pantalone's Pantomime. By David Lord   HMV 7 EG 8981
4. King Monkey. By John Dankworth   HMV 7 EG 8982

Bartók. For Children, and Roumanian Christmas Carols

Grammophon LPM 18272

Roger Fiske. Tunes for Children   HMV 7 EG 8575–6
  A set of two records containing many short pieces for Instrumental Ensemble

Yvonne Adair and John Hosier. Music for Percussion Band (but also suitable for movement)   HMV 7 EG 8656–9
  A set of four records with many short pieces contrasted in style and arranged for instrumental ensemble. (The piano music is available from Boosey and Hawkes.)

Piano Music

Piano music for percussion band arranged or composed by Yvonne Adair:

  Elfin Pranks (Norwegian); The Tinkers by the Stream; Rebel Song (French); Country Dance (Finnish); Court Dance (Danish); The Old Snuff Box (French); Lords and Ladies; Pussy Willow; The Rocking Horse   Boosey and Hawkes
  Mr. Pumphrey   Novello

Folk Dances from Home and Abroad. Parts I and II. Lengnick
Liadov   Eight Russian Folksongs, Op. 58
                             Boosey and Hawkes

Many good examples not included in the list can be found in the standard works of the great composers and among the folk and national songs and dances of all nations. Standard works such as the Bach and Handel suites, Beethoven's Bagatelles, Minuets, and Ecossaises, the smaller piano works of Brahms (Intermezzi, Capriccios), Chopin's Mazurkas, Preludes, Polonaises, and Waltzes, Schubert's Moments Musicaux, Mendelssohn's Songs Without Words, and the vast range of ballet music, can all be obtained from the local library. If the library has no music section it is generally possible for the librarian to get music from other branches. Some Public Libraries are also stocked with recordings of standard works.

4. MUSIC FOR LISTENING

It is a good thing for children to listen to music that they have already danced to, therefore all the music suggested so far will be of use. Additional suggestions of a pictorial kind are given below:

Daquin	Le Coucou
De Severac	Musical Box
Elgar	Wand of Youth: Fairy Pipers and Slumber Scene
Fauré	Dolly Suite: Berceuse
Grainger	Handel in the Strand
Humperdinck	Hansel and Gretel
Kodály	Hâry János: Viennese Musical Clock
Liadov	Eight Russian Folk-Songs: The Gnat (No. 4) Music Box
Mompou	Scènes d'enfants
Perry (Nina)	Through the Kaleidoscope: The Elephant, Donkey, Cowboy Song
Prokofiev	Peter and the Wolf
Quilter	Children's Overture
Respighi	The Birds: The Hen
Rimsky-Korsakov	Flight of the Bumble Bee
Saint-Saëns	Carnival of Animals
Smetana	The Bartered Bride: Dance of the Comedians
Strauss	Thunder and Lightning Polka
Stravinsky	Petrushka: Ballerina's dance
Tchaikovsky	Sleeping Beauty: The Lilac Fairy The Silver Fairy Puss in Boots and the White Cat The Blue Bird Dances Red Riding Hood and the Wolf

Tchaikovsky
The Nutcracker Suite:
Chinese Dance
Dance of the Reed Pipes
Dance of the Sugar Plum Fairy
Spanish Dance

5. THE MARKING OF GRAMOPHONE RECORDS

A yellow chinagraph pencil can be used to mark 78s but not L.Ps. Indeed there is no means of actually marking an L.P. disc. But when the place of a piece of music has been found on the disc it can be noted down by using a strip of cardboard marked out like the following diagram:

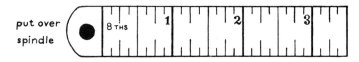

With the use of this 'ruler' the place can be found again quite quickly.

Appendix C

USEFUL MUSICAL TERMS AND MARKS

Accelerando	Getting gradually faster.
Adagio	Slow.
Andante	Flowing—slowish but not slow.
Allargando	Getting slower and slower. Broadening.
Allegro	Quick, lively, bright.
Dolce	Sweet and soft.
Forte (*f*)	Loud.
Fortissimo (*ff*)	Very loud.
Con Grazia	Gracefully.
Largo	Slow and broad.
Larghetto	As for Largo but less so.
Leggiero	Lightly.
Lente	Slow.
Lento	Slow.
Maestoso	Majestically.
Marcato	Marked—each note emphasized.
Piano (*p*)	Soft.
Pianissimo (*pp*)	Very soft.
Presto	Quick.
Prestissimo	Very quick.
Rallentando	Getting gradually slower.
Ritardando	Getting gradually slower.
Ritenuto	Slower.
Stringendo	Quickening the pace.
Vif	Lively.
Vivo	Lively.

Volante		Flying, swift and light.
Vivace		Vivacious.
𝅘𝅥 >	Accent	Note to be played with accentuation.
𝅘𝅥 −	Marked	This note to be marked but less accentuated than the above.
𝅘𝅥 •	Staccato	Note to be played crisply and shortly.
𝄐		Pause. Hold on to the note one beat longer.
		Crescendo. Getting louder.
		Diminuendo. Getting softer.
		Repeat marks. Music within these two signs to be repeated.

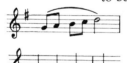

Slur over notes indicates smooth playing or singing

Two notes marked thus indicate a tie. The repeated note is held but not played.

Appendix D

LIST OF MUSIC PUBLISHERS

Name	*Address or English Agent*
Augener	Galliard (see below).
Boosey and Hawkes	295 Regent Street, London, W.1.
Chappell	50 New Bond Street, London, W.1.
Chester	11 Great Marlborough Street, London, W.1.
Choudens	U.M.P. (see below).
Cranz and Co.	Galliard (see below).
Curwen	29 Maiden Lane, London, W.C.2.
Durand	U.M.P. (see below).
Fürstner	Chappell (see above).
Galliard	148 Charing Cross Road, London, W.C.2.
Heugel	U.M.P. (see below).
International Music Co.	509 Fifth Avenue, New York.
Lengnick	160 Wardour Street, London, W.1.
Leduc	U.M.P. (see below).
Macmelodies	21 Denmark Street, London, W.C.2.
Oxford University Press	44 Conduit Street, London, W.1.
Paxton and Co.	36 Dean Street, London, W.1.
Peters, C. F.	Hinrichsen Edition, 10 Baches Street, London, N.1.
Rahter	Novello, 160 Wardour Street, London, W.1.
Schirmer	Chappell (see above).

Schott	48 Great Marlborough Street, London, W.1.
Simrock	Lengnick (see above).
United Music Publishers	1 Montague Street, Russell Square, London, W.C.1.
Universal	2 Fareham Street, London, W.1.

Set and reprinted lithographically by
Ebenezer Baylis & Son Limited
Worcester